Low-Carb Diet

Top 365 Easy to Cook Delicious Low-Carb Diet Mediterranean Recipes for Breakfast, Lunch & Dinner

JAMES ABRAHAM & ALEX DOMENICO

© Copyright 2016 by _____K.M. KASSI_____All rights reserved.

This document is presented with the desire to provide reliable, quality information about the topic in question and the facts discussed within. This eBook is sold under the assumption that neither the author nor the publisher should be asked to provide the services discussed within. If any discussion, professional or legal, is otherwise required a proper professional should be consulted.

This Declaration was held acceptable and equally approved by the Committee of Publishers and Associations as well as the American Bar Association.

The reproduction, duplication or transmission of any of the included information is considered illegal whether done in print or electronically. Creating a recorded copy or a secondary copy of this work is also prohibited unless the action of doing so is first cleared through the Publisher and condoned in writing. All rights reserved.

Any information contained in the following pages is considered accurate and truthful and that any liability through inattention or by any use or misuse of the topics discussed within falls solely on the reader. There are no cases in which the Publisher of this work can be held responsible or be asked to provide reparations for any loss of monetary gain or other damages which may be caused by following the presented information in any way shape or form.

The following information is presented purely for informative purposes and is therefore considered universal. The information presented within is done so without a contract or any other type of assurance as to its quality or validity.

Any trademarks which are used are done so without consent and any use of the same does not imply consent or permission was gained from the owner. Any trademarks or brands found within are purely used for clarification purposes and no owners are in anyway affiliated with this work.

TABLE OF CONTENTS

Introduction..1

Chapter 1 : Mediterranean Low-Carb Breakfast Recipes......................3

Chapter 2 : Mediterranean Low-Carb Lunch Recipes........................29

Chapter 3 : Mediterranean Low-Carb Dinner Recipes........................51

Chapter 4 : Mediterranean Low-Carb Snack Recipes........................96

Conclusion..100

Introduction

This book contains proven steps and strategies on how to prepare 365 easy to cook delicious low-carb Mediterranean recipes.

You will learn fantastic Mediterranean recipes to prepare from breakfast to dinner. They are scrumptious low-carb meals from France, Morocco, Lebanon, Israel, Green and Spain. They all share a common component that makes a Mediterranean dish – legumes, whole grains, wheat, olive oil, chicken, and seafood!

Try the different versions of preparing the classic omelet. Yes, they are one of the easiest meals to prepare using the same ingredients such as ham and cheese. Upgrade your 10 minute meal into a mouthwatering dish you simply cannot resist. Learn how to prepare crepes, quiches, muffins, porridge and more.

True to a good low carb meal, meats (beef, pork and lamb) are included but these are recommended to be moderately eaten. This is to prevent high cholesterol, weight gain and high blood pressure. But you need a hearty lunch to prepare for the entire family! Make their meals (and yours) as exciting as possible with mind-blowing gastronomic flavors. Learn how to prepare these hearty meals in the third chapter.

Dinner time need not be confined to Mac and cheese. Prepare a sumptuous meal that is usually served in the finest Mediterranean restaurants in town. By keeping close to exotic taste of capers, basil and their famous feta cheese, a light meal is up for grabs. Each dish featured in the fourth chapter is carefully planned to have less salt and less sugar.

Food after meal time should not be neglected. In a low-carb diet, you are allowed to eat as much as five small servings. The last chapter will show you the amazing cake and cookie recipes you did not know you still can eat while dieting.

Are you ready chef? Let's start cooking Low-carb Mediterranean meals today! Wish you good luck and thanks again for downloading this book. I hope you enjoy it!

Chapter 1

Mediterranean Low-Carb Breakfast Recipes

Each of the recipes contains good carbohydrates. It has a slow-burn component that is needed to keep you from crashing and wanting sweets after 2 hours.

Category: Crepes, Recipes #1-7

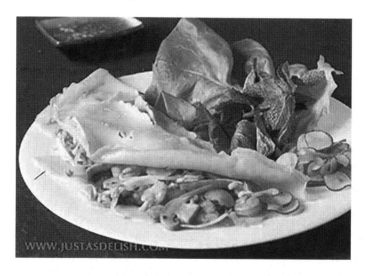

#1 Greek Ricotta and Spinach

Here are the ingredients for you to buy: 1/4 teaspoon minced garlic, 3 tablespoons fat-free ricotta cheese, 2 tablespoons olive oil, Pepper (to taste), 1/4 cup frozen spinach and 1 cup almond milk.

To make this dish, heat the olive oil and sauté the garlic and spinach leaves in a skillet. Add the almond milk and ricotta cheese; mix well. Flip the crepe in half and serve immediately. Garnish with parsley and enjoy!

#2 Spinach Crepes in Romano Cheese

Variation #1; replace Greek ricotta with Romano cheese.

#3 Asparagus Crepes in Romano Cheese

Variation #2; replace spinach with ¼ cup asparagus.

#4 Plantain in Organic Honey

1 large green plantain, 3 eggs, 2 tablespoons extra virgin coconut oil, 3 tablespoon water, and 1 organic honey.

In a food processor or a blender, blend all ingredients. Grease a crepe maker with coconut oil; add pureed mixture and chopped plantain. In a pan, spread the batter and cook for a minute on one side and another minute on the other. Put a dollop of organic honey on top.

#5 Banana in Organic Honey Crepes

Variation #1; replace plantain with 1 large banana.

#6 Ham, Scallions and Arugula

Create this recipe by preparing 12 crêpes (store-bought), 1 bunch arugula, 12 slices lean ham (1/2 inch thick), ½ cup cream cheese (reduced-fat), 2 scallions, and 2 tablespoons milk (fat-free).

Make this dish by whisking milk, scallions and cream cheese in a small bowl. Cook it faster by using a pressure cooker and setting it to 20 minutes on high. Get one crêpe and spread the cream cheese mixture, ham and arugula; roll crêpe. Repeat the process for all 12 rolls and serve the crepes.

#7 Bacon and Arugula Crepe

Variation #1; replace ham with 12 slices bacon.

Category: Omelets, Recipes #8-29

Eggs can be cooked in different ways such as scrambled, omelet, frittata, crepe and egg casseroles. What is in a name, you may ask. Just rich protein content for your low-carb diet, that's for sure. Here are more ways than one to prepare your morning meals.

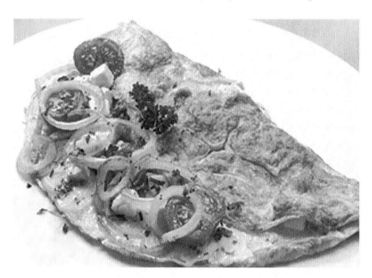

#8 Ultimate Omelet Au Fromage

To create this low carb omelet, prepare 3 tarragon leaves (chopped), 6 tbsp. unsalted butter, 3 tbsp. ricotta cheese, 1 tbsp. parsley, 3 eggs, 1 tsp. Parmesan cheese, and 1 tbsp. chives.

Prepare it by adding butter and add 3 eggs in a pan; add Parmesan and pepper. Tilt the pan back and forth to create an omelet. Fold the omelet in half; add the remaining unsalted butter. Serve your classic cheese omelet on a plate and garnish with parsley.

#9 Double Layered Provençal Omelet

To make this dish for 4 people, prepare 3 cups ricotta cheese, 1 red chili (no seeds), 1 garlic clove, 10 eggs, 2 zucchinis, 4 roasted red peppers (stored-bought), 2 tbsp. fresh basil, 3 spring onions, 6 tbsp. low fat milk, 4 tbsp. chives and olive oil (for drizzling and frying).

Start putting them together by breaking 5 eggs in a bowl and season with pepper. In another bowl, break the remaining eggs and season as well; stir in the roasted peppers and chili. In a skillet, add the chopped zucchini, spring onions in olive oil; sauté for 10 minutes. In a pan, heat olive oil and pour the zucchini-egg mixture. Transfer omelet on a plate; set aside. In the same pan, cook the roasted pepper and chili egg mixture with olive oil. Put the cooked omelet on top of the zucchini omelet. In a bowl, add soft cheese, milk, pepper, and the remaining herbs. Line a cake tin with cling film and add the roasted pepper omelet. Spread a thin layer of the cheese mixture; cover with the zucchini omelet. Serve a slice on a plate and garnish with arugula on top.

#10 Zucchini-Turmeric and Ricotta Frittatas

This dish is a big hit for its low carbohydrates. Set in the Mediterranean group of countries who else can go wrong with a filling treat? Prepare 1 lb. zucchini, 4 eggs, 2 medium onions, 5 garlic cloves, 1/3 cup light ricotta cheese, vegetable oil (for frying), 1/2 tsp. turmeric, and pepper (to taste).

Begin by sautéing onions, turmeric and garlic in a pan. Add grated zucchini and sauté until cooked. In a small bowl, add 4 eggs, ricotta cheese and season with pepper. Drain the zucchini and mix with the eggs. Transfer the zucchini mixture to a baking dish and bake for 30 minutes at 375 degrees F. Once done, serve the baked frittata on a plate and eat it while hot.

#11 Bacon and Turnip Frittata

6 strips of chopped bacon, bacon fat (for frying), 1 lb. turnip, 8 pieces of minced baby bellas, 2 leeks (washed and sliced), Nutmeg (a pinch), 1 can of coconut milk, 4 pieces of scallions, and 1/4 teaspoon ground black pepper.

Cook the bacon strips in a non-stick pan; set aside. Shred the turnips and transfer them in a mixing bowl. Add the reserved bacon fat and combine it with black pepper, nutmeg, salt, leeks, and coconut milk. Transfer the turnip mixture to a 2 quart dish. Top the turnip mixture with bacon, baby bellas and scallions. Bake for one hour at 350 degrees F.

#12 Parsnip Frittata with Crunchy Duck Strips

6 strips of chopped duck meat, duck fat (for frying), 1 lb. parsnips, 8 pieces of minced baby bellas, 2 leeks (washed and sliced), Nutmeg (a pinch), 1 can of coconut milk, 4 pieces of scallions, and 1/4 teaspoon ground black pepper.

Cook the duck strips in a non-stick pan; set aside. Shred the parsnips; transfer to a mixing bowl. Add the reserved duck fat and combine it with black pepper, nutmeg, kosher salt, leeks, and coconut milk. Transfer the parsnips mixture to a baking dish. Top the parsnip mixture with crunchy duck strips, baby bellas and scallions. Bake for one hour at 350 degrees F and serve when done.

#13 Parsnip Frittata with Crunchy Duck Strips

Variation #1; replace turnips with 1 lb. parsnips.

#14 Potato-Zucchini, and Mushroom Omelet

1 small zucchini, 5 small potatoes, 5 medium mushrooms , 5 egg whites , vegetable cooking spray, 3 ounces mozzarella cheese,

pepper to taste, ½ medium onions, 3 whole eggs, 1 tbsp. parmesan cheese, and 1 ½ cups red bell peppers.

In a pot, boil water and cook the potatoes until tender. Grease a pan with vegetable cooking spray and sauté the onions. Add the zucchini, red peppers and mushrooms; sauté until tender. In a large bowl, mix the egg whites, garlic salt, pepper, eggs and mozzarella cheese. Toss the vegetables with the egg white mixture and set aside. Meanwhile, grease a large skillet with vegetable cooking spray; pour the egg white mixture, potatoes and parmesan cheese. Bake for 30 minutes at 375 degrees F.

Remove the omelet from the oven and allow it to cool for about 10 minutes. Slice the omelet and serve on individual plates; garnish with parsley and enjoy!

#15 Potato-Asparagus, and Mushroom Omelet

Variation #1, replace zucchini with 2 asparagus bunches.

#16 Potato-Arugula, and Mushroom Omelet

Variation #2, replace zucchini with 2 pieces arugula bunches.

#17 Salmon Scrambled Eggs with Sour Cream Dip

1 piece smoked salmon, 1/3 cup milk (fat-free), 1 small red onion, 8 tablespoons sour cream (reduced-fat), 2 teaspoons olive oil, ¼ teaspoon black pepper, 1 egg, and 2 tablespoons fresh dill.

Prepare it by adding vegetable oil in a skillet to sauté the onions until soft; set aside. In a medium-sized bowl, combine the fat-free milk, egg, salmon and pepper. In the same skillet, add the salmon mixture and scramble the eggs until set. Serve on a plate and add a dollop of sour cream and a sprinkle of dill.

#18 Tuna Scrambles in Sour Cream

Variation #1; replace salmon with 1 piece smoked tuna.

#19 Scrambled Eggs with smoked Halibut

Variation #2; replace salmon with 1 piece smoked halibut

#20 Crab Omelet with Celery and Onions

You need the right ingredients to make you full and full of energy. All you have to do is prepare 1 tablespoon chopped celery, 4 eggs, 3/4 cup crabmeat, 1 tablespoon minced onion, and 2 tablespoons unsalted butter.

Cook it by beating 4 eggs and cooking it in a pan over medium heat. Sauté the minced onions in butter and add the crabmeat and celery; simmer for about 3 minutes. Spread the crabmeat mixture on the omelet and fold it in half. Serve on a plate and garnish it with parsley.

#21 Shrimp Omelet with Celery and Onions

Variation #1; replace the crabmeat with ½ cup shrimps.

#22 Eggs in Sugar Snap Peas and Spinach

2 tablespoons olive oil, 1/2 leek (thinly sliced), 2 cups sugar snap peas, 2 cups spinach leaves (chopped), Pepper (to taste), and 2 eggs.

In a skillet, add olive oil and sauté the leeks for 5 minutes. Add the sugar snap peas and spinach; cook until slightly wilted. Add pepper to taste. Arrange spinach mixture, create a well in the middle; crack the eggs. Cook eggs for 6 minutes. To serve, transfer to a plate and enjoy!

#23 Asparagus and Sugar Snap Peas Omelet

Variation #1; replace the spinach with 1 bunch of asparagus.

#24 Hominy, Bacon and Eggs Mornings

1 can hominy (maize kernels), 4 eggs, ¼ pound sliced bacon, ¼ cup chopped onion, and 1/4 teaspoon pepper.

In a skillet, add onions and bacon; cook until the bacon is crispy and onions are tender. Stir in pepper, beaten eggs and hominy; cook until eggs are set. Serve warm on a plate.

#25 Kernel Corns and Bacon Omelet

Variation #1; replace the hominy with 1 can of kernel corns.

#26 Eggxiting Kernel Bacon

Variation #2; replace the kernel corn with ½ can cream-style corn.

#27 Tuna-Filled Scrambled Egg with Aioli

1 cup plain yogurt, pepper to taste, 1 tbsp. lemon juice, 7 eggs, small handful of basil, Garlic powder (to taste), and 1 can tuna in water (drained).

In a medium-sized pot, boil the eggs with water; allow them to cool down before setting aside. In a small bowl, mix garlic powder, basil, lemon juice, pepper, yogurt, and tuna. In a plate, cut eggs in half and scoop out the yolk. Mix the yolk with the prepared mixture and place the tuna into the emptied eggs. Serve on a plate and garnish with a basil leaf.

#28 Salmon-Filled Scrambles with Aioli

Variation #1; replace the 1 can of tuna with 1 can of salmon.

#29 Shrimp-Filled Scrambles with Aioli

Variation #2; replace the 1 can of tuna and salmon with ½ cup shrimps.

Category: Muffins, Recipe #30-36

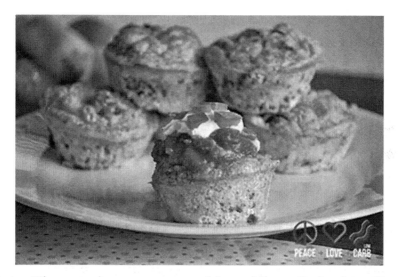

Note: These recipes are prepared by adding all the ingredients together in bowl. Prepare a muffin pan and pour the batter. Bake in the over at 400 degrees F for 20 minutes. Once done, remove the muffins from the pan and serve immediately.

#30 Apple-Cinnamon Mini Muffins with Ricotta Cheese

Muffins are great in the morning so head on to your pantry and take 1 tbsp. vanilla extract, 1 tsp. baking soda, 1 cup low-fat buttermilk, 3 tbsp. cane sugar, 1 tbsp. baking powder, 3 tbsp. vegetable oil, cooking spray, 1 large egg, 2 tsp. ground cinnamon, 2 large egg whites, 1 1/2 cups apple, 2 tsp. ground cinnamon, 1/3 cup light ricotta cheese, and 2 cups all-purpose flour.

#31 Cinnamon Mini Muffins with Pears an Ricotta Cheese

Variation #1; replace the apples with 1 ½ cups fresh pear.

#32 Parma Ham with Broccoli and Bell Pepper Crumpets

1 small bunch of spinach, ¼ cup sliced and diced mushrooms, 6 slices Parma ham (slice into 4 strips), 1/2 cup broccoli, 12 eggs, cooking spray (vegetable oil), 1 small bell pepper and raw honey (for topping).

#33 Bacon and Broccoli Egg Crumpets

Variation #1, replace Parma ham with 10 bacon strips.

#34 Cinnamon Bran Cereal Muffin with Crushed Pineapple

To make this recipe, you need 1 can crushed pineapple, 3/4 cup milk (fat-free), 1 cup shredded carrot, 1 teaspoon ground cinnamon, 1 cup wheat bran flakes cereal, 1 teaspoon baking soda, 1 and 3/4 cups all-purpose flour, cooking spray, 2 tablespoons butter, 2 tablespoons water, 1/4 cup cane sugar, 1 teaspoon baking powder, and1 large egg.

#35 Mushroom-Broccoli Bacon Muffins

Get 6 cooked bacon, 1/2 cup broccoli, 12 eggs, 1 small bell pepper, 1 small bunch of spinach, and ¼ cup diced mushrooms.

#36 Zucchini-Lemon Muffins

All you have to do is prepare 2 teaspoons grated lemon rind, 1 cup coarsely shredded zucchini, 3/4 cup skim milk, 2 cups coconut flour, 1 egg, 1/4 teaspoon ground nutmeg, ¼ cup cane sugar, and cooking spray.

Category: Quiche, Recipe #37-44

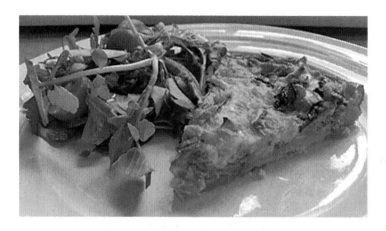

#37 Pimiento, Ham and Swiss cheese Quiche

For this delicious recipe, you will need 1/2 lb. cooked ham, 4 teaspoons all-purpose flour, 1 cup non-fat milk, 2 tablespoons pimento peppers (for garnishing), 1 9-inch frozen pie whole-wheat crust, 1/4 teaspoon dry mustard, 2 tablespoons parsley (for garnishing), 3 eggs, and 1 1/2 cups grated Swiss cheese.

To make the dish, add grated Swiss cheese with the all-purpose. When fully combined, dust the cheese and flour mixture on the pie shell. Sprinkle mixture into the pie shell and top it with ham and the remaining cheese. In a medium bowl, combine the mustard powder, heavy cream, and eggs. Mix all the ingredients and pour the smooth batter over the ham and cheese. Place the quiche muffin pan on top of the trivet and set the pressure cooker to 25 minutes over high heat. Garnish with chopped pimiento pepper and chopped parsley then serve.

#38 Bacon and Zucchini-Spinach Quiche

You need 2 pieces of organic zucchini (grated), 1 1/2 tablespoon coconut flour, 1 egg, 1 tablespoon of coconut oil, and 1 teaspoon flax meal. For the quiche, you will need 1/2 cup organic egg whites, 1/4 teaspoon ground mustard seeds, 5 eggs (beaten), 3 tablespoon of almond milk, 1/2 cup fresh spinach (chopped), and 5 slices bacon. For the topping, you will need 1/2 cup cheese (grated), and 2 tomatoes (sliced).

To begin, preheat the oven to 400 degrees F and grease a pie dish with olive oil. Add drained grated zucchini, coconut flour, egg, coconut oil, and flax meal. Evenly spread on the pie dish and bake for 9 minutes. In a large bowl, mix the egg whites, ground mustard, eggs, and milk. Add chopped spinach and chopped bacon to the egg mixture. Pour the prepared egg mixture into the zucchini crust. Place the tomato slices on top and bake for about 28 minutes. Remove from the oven and let it cool down. Slice the quiche and serve with tomato slices on top.

#39 Cheesy Baby Spinach Bacon Quiche

To make this recipe, you will need 1 pie crust, 6 eggs, 1 lb. bacon, 1 1/2 cups heavy cream, 1 1/2 cups Swiss cheese, pepper, and 2 cups baby spinach leaves.

Use a food processor to combine the pepper, cream, eggs, pepper and salt. Prepare a 9 inch pie crust; put the cheese, spinach and bacon. In a medium bowl, whisk 6 large eggs and pour on top of the pie crust. Put the pie crust on a glass pie plate and bake in the oven for about 35 minutes at 375 degrees F. Once done, slice into wedges and serve.

#40 Baby Spinach and Asparagus Quiche

Variation #1; replace spinach with1 bunch of asparagus.

#41 "Ham and Swiss" Quiche

1/2 cup cooked ham, 4 tsp. all-purpose flour, 1 cup almond milk, 2 tbsp. pimento peppers (for garnishing), 1 pie crust, 1/4 tsp. dry mustard, 2 tbsp. parsley (for garnishing), 3 eggs, and 1 1/2 cups grated Swiss cheese.

Here's how to do it. In medium bowl, mix the grated Swiss cheese with the all-purpose. When fully combined dust the cheese and flour mixture on the pie shell. Sprinkle mixture into the pie shell and top it with ham and the remaining of the cheese. In medium bowl, combine the mustard powder, heavy cream, and eggs. Mix all the ingredients and pour the smooth batter over the ham and cheese. Bake it in the oven for about an hour at 400 degrees F. To serve, garnish with chopped pimiento peppers and chopped parsley.

#42 2-Cheese Spinach Quiche

1 pie crust, 10 oz. package frozen spinach, 1 cup milk, 1/2 cup unsalted butter, 1 small onion, 3 cloves garlic, 1 package herb and garlic feta, 1 can mushrooms,1 block Cheddar cheese, 4 eggs, and pepper to taste.

In a medium skillet, melt butter and sauté onion and garlic for 7 minutes. Stir in fat cheese, mushrooms and cheddar cheese. Spoon the mixture on a pastry shell and season it with pepper. In a medium bowl, mix pepper, milk and salt with beaten eggs. Pour the egg mixture into the shell and combine with the thawed spinach leaves. Line the pastry shells on a baking tray; bake in the oven for 15 minutes at 375 degrees F. Serve in mini plates and enjoy while hot.

#43 2-cheese Asparagus Quiche

Variation #1; replace spinach with 5 bunches of asparagus stalks.

#44 2-cheese Arugula Quiche

Variation #2; replace spinach with 5 bunches of arugula leaves.

Category: Porridge, Recipe #45-56

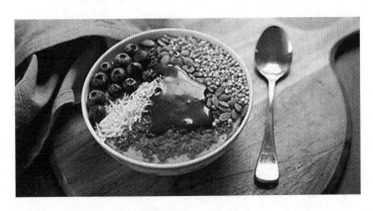

#45 Almond and Coconut Flaxseed Porridge

You will need 1 tbsp. Flaxseed Meal , ½ cup hot water, ¼ cup almonds (sliced), ¼ cup shredded coconut (unsweetened), 2 tbsp. shelled pumpkin seeds (raw), ½ tbsp. Honey (to taste), and ¼ cup Walnuts (raw). In a food processor or blender, mix the walnuts, flaxseed, coconut, almonds and pumpkin seeds.

In a microwavable dish, add water, honey and oil. Microwave for 30 seconds; set aside to allow the porridge to cool and thicken.

#46 Nutmeg-Cinnamon Flaxseed

Variation #1; just add ½ tsp. ground nutmeg and ½ tsp. ground cinnamon.

#47 Flaxseed, Cinnamon and Apple Crisper

Variation #2; just add ½ tsp. cinnamon and 2 tbsp. dried apples.

#48 Pecan-Maple Flaxseed

Variation #3; just add 2 tbsp. chopped pecan and 1 tbsp. raw honey.

#49 Pecan-Banana Flaxseed

Variation #4; just add 2 tbsp. pecan slivers and 1 banana.

#50 Flaxseed and Creamy Peaches

Variation #5; just ½ fresh peaches (chopped), and 2 tbsp. heavy cream.

#51 Pumpkin in Cinnamon and Ginger Flaxseed

Variation #6; just add 1/4 tsp. ground ginger, 1/4 tsp. ground cinnamon, 1/4 tsp. ground cloves, 1/4 tsp. ground allspice, 1/4 tsp. ground nutmeg, and ¼ cup pumpkin puree. Add them to the base porridge ingredients and serve hot.

#52 Salty Butter-Flaxseed

Variation #7; just add 2 tbsp. unsalted butter, and ½ tsp. Himalayan sea salt.

#53 Cocoa-Flaxseed

Variation #8; just add 1 tbsp. cocoa powder with the rest of the ingredients.

#54 Pecan-Coconut Flaxseed Porridge

Variation #9; just add ¼ cup pecan slivers and ½ tsp. ground cinnamon.

#55 Flaxseed, Cinnamon and Mango Crisper

Variation #10; just add ½ tsp. cinnamon and 2 tbsp. chopped dried mangoes.

#56 Homemade Oatmeal with Nuts and Spices

1 teaspoon ground cloves, 1 cup chopped dried dates, 2 tablespoons ground cinnamon, 1 cup chopped walnuts, 1 cup brown sugar, 1 teaspoon ground turmeric, 1 cup chopped dried apples, 3 cups grain cereal flakes, 1 tablespoon ground ginger, and 3 cups rolled oats. Make it by combining dates, oats, cereal, walnuts, apples, brown sugar, cloves, turmeric and ginger in a large bowl.

In a microwave, boil one cup of water and pour it over the large bowl. Stir the oatmeal mix and make sure every dry ingredient is softened and let it stand for 10 minutes before serving.

Category: Pancakes, Recipe #57-64

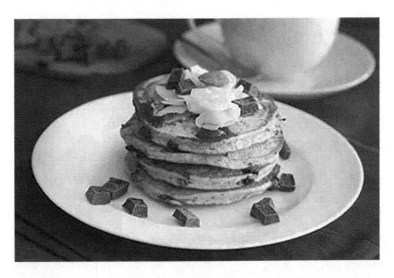

#57 Blueberries in Buttermilk Pancakes

You need 1 1/4 cups buttermilk (low-fat), 1 cup almond flour, 1 tablespoon cane sugar, 1 tablespoon vegetable oil, 1 egg, cooking spray, 1/2 cup frozen blueberries and raw maple syrup (for topping).

To cook it, you will need a large bowl to combine the almond flour and cane sugar. Add in the egg, oil and buttermilk to the dry ingredients, stir in blueberries. Coat a skillet with cooking spray and pour ¼ cup of the batter. Transfer into a plate and drizzle maple syrup; serve with blueberries on the side.

#58 Raspberry-Buttermilk Pancakes

Variation #1; replace the blueberries with ½ cup raspberries.

#59 Strawberry-Buttermilk Pancakes

Variation #2; replace the blueberries with ½ cup strawberries.

#60 Blackberry-Buttermilk Pancakes

Variation #3; replace the blueberries with ½ cup blackberries.

#61 Corn Kernel-Buttermilk Pancakes

Variation #4; replace the blueberries with ½ can of kernel corn.

#62 Sweet Potato with Nutmeg Breakfast Cakes

Sweet potatoes are the best alternative for a low carb meal. That is why you need to prepare this recipe that has the following ingredients: 1 lb. sweet potato, 1 teaspoon onion, 1 egg, 1 teaspoons ground nutmeg, pepper (to taste), 1/4 cup coconut flour, and cooking spray.

Start cooking by combining peeled and shredded sweet potatoes, coconut flour, pepper, egg and nutmeg. In a large skillet, grease with cooking spray and add all the ingredients; cook for about four minutes. Flatten the cooked sweet potatoes and constantly stir until golden brown. Serve on a plate and enjoy!

#63 Banana-Cashew and Almond Pancakes

4 pieces bananas (ripe), 1/2 cup almond, 2 tsp. olive oil, 4 pieces organic eggs, ½ cup cashew, and black pepper to taste.

Combine mashed bananas and pre-beaten eggs in a large bowl. Add the cashews and almonds and mix well until smooth and creamy. Season the batter with black pepper. In a small skillet, add ¼ cup of the pancake batter and cook with olive oil. Flip each side until golden brown; serve with raw honey.

#64 Banana-Macadamia and Almond Pancakes

Variation #1; replace the cashews with ½ cup macadamia nuts.

Category: Low-carb Bread, Recipe #65-71

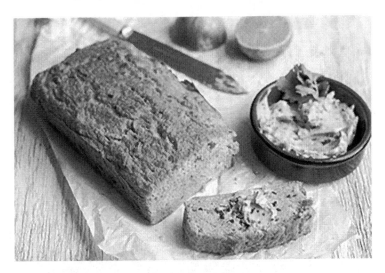

#65 Coconut Rosemary Nut-Free Bread

4 eggs, 1/4 cup coconut milk, 1/4 cup olive oil, 1 teaspoon baking soda, 1/3 cup flax meal, 1 teaspoon freshly ground rosemary, and 3/4 cup coconut flour.

Preheat your oven to 350 degrees F. In a bowl, beat eggs with a hand mixer. In a medium-sized bowl, add coconut milk, flax meal, baking soda, olive oil, sea salt and rosemary. Sift the coconut flour and add to the mixture; bake for 45 minutes. Allow it to cool before serving.

#66 Oven-Baked Coconut Cheesy Bread

You need 1/4 cup Romano cheese, 2 cups Tapioca flour, 1/4 cup coconut oil, 1/4 cup coconut milk, and 2 eggs. Preheat your oven to 450 degrees F.

In a medium-sized bowl, mix dry and wet ingredients. Transfer to a cookie sheet and knead the dough. Brush coconut oil over the dough and sprinkle grated Romano cheese. Place the dough in the oven and bake for 15 minutes. Serve immediately.

#67 Yellow Cornbread Muffins

1 tablespoon baking powder, 1 egg, 1 cup all-purpose flour, 3 tablespoons cane sugar, 2 cups yellow cornmeal, 1 and 1/2 cups milk, and 1/3 cup vegetable oil.

Preheat your oven to 425 degrees F and grease a muffin tin with cooking spray. In a medium-sized bowl, add the oil, milk, egg, cornmeal, all-purpose flour, baking powder, and sugar; combine well. Spoon the batter into the tin muffins and bake for 20 minutes. Remove muffins from the muffin tins and serve them warm with butter on top.

#68 Spicy Cornmeal Blueberry Bread

This is variation #1. Add 1 tsp. cayenne pepper and 5 cups blueberries to the list of ingredients.

#69 Grilled Multi-grain Bread with Zucchini and Olive-Yogurt Dressing

½ cup plain yogurt, ¼ cup basil leaves, 1 small zucchini, 4 sliced hard cheese, 8 slices whole grain bread, 1 jar red roasted peppers, and 2 tsp. black olives (chopped).

To prepare the salad, combine the plain yogurt with the chopped black olives in a bowl. Take a slice of wholegrain bread, spread the mixture and top with hard cheese, zucchini, bacon bits and peppers. To make this meal more interesting, heat a pan, add olive oil and place the bread on top. Add a slice of cheese on the bread, flip it until it melts. Serve right away and enjoy!

#70 Banana Bread with Cinnamon and Almonds

You need 4 bananas, 2 cups cane sugar, 1 tablespoon baking soda, ½ cups of almonds, 1 cup almond milk, ½ cup vegetable oil, 3 teaspoons cinnamon, 4 medium eggs, and 4 cups of almond flour.

Combine the first 4 ingredients and blend in mixer for 1 minute; transfer to a bowl. Mix the oil, almond milk, almond flour, almonds and eggs. In a greased loaf pan, pour the batter and sprinkle cinnamon on top. Bake at 275 degrees F for 2 and ½ hours. Once the bread is done, allow it to cool for 5 minutes before serving.

#71 Banana Bread with Cinnamon and Pecan Slivers

Variation #1; replace almonds with 1 cup pecan slivers.

Category: Breakfast Smoothies, Recipe #72-93

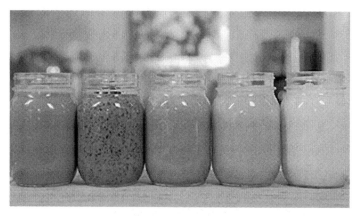

Note: for the directions, all smoothies are prepared the same way. Unless otherwise stated that ingredients require cooking before being blended. Prepare a thirst-quenching and satisfying smoothie by adding the ingredients to a blender. Set the timer to 30 seconds and puree until smooth. Pour contents into a tall glass or Mason jar and serve.

#72 Strawberry-Banana Flaxseed Smoothie

2 tbsp. flaxseed meal, 1 cup almond milk (unsweetened), ½ piece of banana, 5 ice cubes, 1 cup strawberries, and raw honey (to taste).

#73 Banana-Carrot Smoothie

½ cup baby carrots, 1 cup cold almond milk (unsweetened), 1 banana, ½ tsp. vanilla extract, raw honey (to taste), and 2 tbsp. flaxseed meal.

#74 Cherry-Almond Milk Smoothie

½ cup yogurt, 1 cup almond milk (unsweetened), 1 cup frozen cherries, raw honey (to taste), and 5 ice cubes.

#75 Low-Carb Papaya-Almond Smoothie

Raw honey (to taste), 1/3 cup almond milk, 2 cups papaya juice, 1 small ripe papaya, and 6 ice cubes.

#76 Avocado Smoothie with Yogurt and Green Tea

1/2 cup plain yogurt, raw honey (to taste), 1 1/4 cup unsweetened almond milk, 1 tbsp. water, 1 tsp. green tea powder, and 1/2 medium avocado.

#77 Berry Spinach-Chia Smoothie

1 tsp. ground cinnamon, 2 cups spinach, 1/4 cup chia seeds, 1/2 cup strawberries, 2 tbsp. walnuts (chopped), 1/2 cup blueberries, cinnamon powder (for garnishing), 2 cups water (for softening the chia seeds), and 1 tbsp. ground flax seed.

Prior to blending the ingredients, you need to soften the chia seeds. Do this by soaking the chia seeds in bowl of hot water. Leave the bowl covered for 30 minutes until seeds soften and soaks up the water. Transfer to a blender and puree as instructed.

#78 Blueberry-Almond Smoothie

2 tbsp. almond milk, 1 1/2 cup fresh blueberries, 1/2 cup Greek yogurt (fat-free), 1/4 cup almonds (slivers), 2 tsp. raw honey, cinnamon powder (for garnishing), and 1 cup ice cubes.

#79 Strawberry-Banana Yogurt Smoothie

1 cup strawberry yogurt (sugar-free), 2 cups crushed ice, 1 cup fresh strawberries, and 1 banana.

#80 Orange, Soy Milk and Banana

1 banana, 1/2 cup of orange juice, 1 cup fortified soy milk, and 2 cups crushed ice.

#81 Peanut Butter Festive Latte in Dark Choco-Vanilla

1 cup almond milk, 2 cups coffee cubes*, ¼ cup dark chocolate syrup, 2 tbsp. peanut butter, and 2 tsp. vanilla extract.

Prepare the coffee cubes* at least 2 hours before making the latte. Brew strong coffee, once cool, pour into ice trays; freeze.

#82 Apple-Almond and Ginger Yogurt Smoothie

½ cup low-fat yogurt, 1 apple, 1 tsp. cinnamon, 1 cup almond milk (unsweetened), and 5 almonds.

#83 Peach-Banana Almond Milk Smoothie

1 grated ginger, 1 small banana, ¼ teaspoon vanilla extract, 1 cup peaches, and 1 cup cold almond milk.

#84 Chia and Apple-Avocado

1/2 cup of skim milk, 2 tbsp. chia seeds, 1/2 avocado, 1/2 cup fresh pineapple cubes, 1/2 apple, 1/2 cup broccoli, 1/2 cup of spinach leaves, and 1 cup ice.

#85 Vanilla Milk in Apple and Banana

½ cored apple, 1 tsp. cinnamon, Stevia (to taste), 1 1/2 cup vanilla almond milk (unsweetened), and 1 banana.

#86 Apricot-Vanilla Swirl

1 tbsp. agave syrup, 10 apricots (dried), 1 cup vanilla almond milk (unsweetened), and ½ cup plain yogurt.

#87 Strawberry-Banana Flaxseed

Add agave syrup (to taste), 1 cup cold almond milk (unsweetened), 1 cup of fresh strawberries, and 1 banana.

#88 Banana-Carrot Flaxseed

½ cup baby carrots, 1 cup cold almond milk (unsweetened), 1 banana, ½ tsp. vanilla extract, Stevia (to taste).

#89 Creamy Cherry-Chocolate

½ cup yogurt, 1 cup cold chocolate almond milk (unsweetened), 2 cups cherries, 1 tbsp. raw honey, and 5 ice cubes.

#90 Papaya Smoothie in Skim Milk and Honey

1 tbsp. raw honey, 1/4 cup skim milk, 2 cups papaya juice, 1 small ripe papaya, and 6 ice cubes.

#91 Avocado Power Yogurt Smoothie with Green Tea

1/2 cup plain yogurt, 2 tsp. Stevia, 1 1/4 cup unsweetened almond milk,, 1 tbsp. hot water, 1 tsp. green tea powder, and 1/2 medium avocado.

#91 Kale-Strawberry-Lime Smoothie

2 tsp. grated ginger, 1 1/2 cups of fresh strawberries, 6 large kale leaves, 2 tsp. raw honey, 3 tbsp. lime juice, and 1/2 cup cold water.

#92 Cabbage Power Smoothie with Apples and Citrus

1 apple, 1 orange, ½ cabbage, 1/2 lemon, 1 cup water, and 2 cups ice cubes.

#93 Fruity Spinach and Ginger Smoothie

You need 2 medium carrots, 1 medium apple, 2 bundles baby spinach, 1 tbsp. ginger root, and 2 cups water.

Category: Sausages, Recipe #94-96

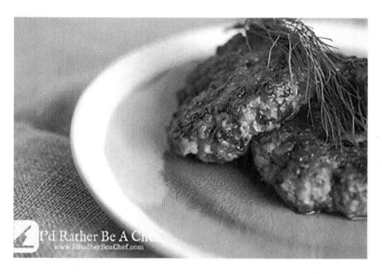

#94 Breakfast Sausages in Rosemary and Olive Oil

To prepare this dish, you need 1 package breakfast sausages, 1 tablespoon olive oil, 1 teaspoon fresh rosemary, 1 medium onion, fresh rosemary sprigs (for garnishing) 2 teaspoons whole grain mustard, and freshly ground black pepper.

To cook it, preheat your oven to 500 degrees F and prepare an ungreased baking sheet. In a small skillet, sauté chopped rosemary leaves, onions in olive oil; set aside in a bowl. In the same skillet, add ground pepper, mustard and sausages with casings. Mix the sausage mixture and form into patties; transfer to a baking sheet and bake for 6 minutes. Remove to blot excess oil and garnish the breakfast sausages with rosemary sprigs and serve.

#95 Corned Beef with Potatoes and Over-Easy Eggs

You will need 2 tablespoons vegetable oil, 4 slices cheddar cheese, 4 tablespoons unsalted butter, 1 bell pepper, 4 large eggs, 1 white onion, 8 ounces corned beef, 2 medium baking potatoes, and pepper (to taste).

In a skillet, cook bell pepper, potatoes, onions and corned beef. Stir the contents until the potatoes turn golden brown. In another skillet, add butter and fry eggs over-easy; season with pepper; set aside. Place cheese over the corned beef and let cheese melt for a minute. Serve on a plate and top with the eggs over-easy.

#96 Potato Hash with Crumbled Sausages

For this dish, you will need 8 0unces Italian sausage (hot), 2 tablespoons parsley, 3 tablespoons unsalted butter, a dash of hot sauce, 3 tablespoons olive oil (extra virgin), 1 1/4 lbs. baking potatoes, 4 ounces Italian sausage (mild) and black pepper (to taste)

For your potato hash you need to add the peeled potatoes in a bowl; set aside. In a large pan, add olive oil and fry crumbled sausages; cook for 12 minutes. Transfer sausages to paper towels to drain excess oil. Place the sausages back in the pan, add butter and olive oil; sauté the potatoes and season with pepper. When potatoes turn lightly brown, add the sausages and chopped parsley; remove from heat. Serve on a dish and add a dash of hot sauce to enjoy!

Chapter 2

Mediterranean Low-Carb Lunch Recipes

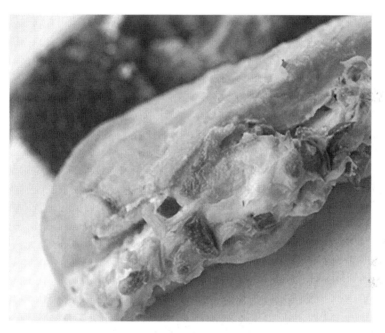

Did you know that a large pita has only 25 grams of carbohydrates? In the succeeding recipes, 2 pitas mean two people can share. This segment will give you fish, chicken, turkey, and beef low-carb recipes. There are a lot to choose from so you will not run out of ideas.

Category: Chicken, Recipe #97-126

#97 Chicken in Saffron Butter

You need 2 tbsp. fresh squeezed lemon, 1 tbsp. saffron, 4 tbsp. butter, 12 whole chicken wings, cooking spray (vegetable oil), pepper (to taste), and 3 lemon wedges (for garnishing).

To cook it you need a steamer basket. Place the chicken and steam for 10 minutes. In a small pan, melt butter and pour the saffron; set aside. Prepare a cookie sheet; line with parchment paper. Arrange chicken on the sheet; lightly spray with vegetable oil. Bake for 30 minutes at 425 degrees F. Serve chicken on a large plate and pour the saffron butter on top and garnish with lemon wedges.

#98 Slow-cooked Chicken Breasts in Rosemary

For this 3-ingredient Mediterranean meal, you need 1/2 cup of dried rosemary leaves, 1 bottle Italian dressing, and 5 pieces boneless chicken breasts.

Get a crockpot to cook the chicken. Add rosemary and the Italian dressing together. Set heat to 4 hours over high heat. Once timer is up, serve chicken on a plate and enjoy.

#99 Low Carb Italian Chicken Breasts with Light Cream Cheese

Another variation of your slow-cook Mediterranean meal, you need 1 package light cream cheese, 4 chicken breasts, and a packet of Italian seasoning.

All you have to do is combine chicken breasts, seasoning, and light cream cheese in slow cooker. Cook for 4 hours on high heat. Once done, you may serve dish on a plate of freshly cooked pasta.

#100 Mediterranean Chicken over Lettuce and Fruits

This recipe needs 1 cup strawberries, 1 cup peaches, ½ cup non-fat yogurt, ½ cup celery, ½ cup pineapple chunks, 2 tbsp. mint, 4 cups lettuce, ½ tsp. lemon rind, ½ tsp. cinnamon, and 2 oz. chicken breast.

You will need a bowl to combine the celery and fruits. In a separate bowl, add cinnamon, yogurt, mint and lemon rind; mix to combine and pour over chicken. Transfer the fruits and celery before serving. In individual bowls, place lettuce and scoop the salad on top.

#101 Cheddar and Chicken with Sweet Potatoes

For a slow-cooked recipe, you need 1 package of cheddar cheese, 4 chicken breasts (skinless), 3 sweet potatoes wedges, and 1 packet of Italian seasoning.

Mix the chicken breasts, potato wedges, seasoning and cheddar cheese in a slow cooker and cook for 4 hours on high heat. Serve on a plate and enjoy the succulent treat.

#102 Peppered Chicken Roast with Garlic and Paprika

1 lb. whole chicken, 2 tbsp. black pepper, 2 tbsp. paprika, 2 tbsp. garlic powder. The direction for this meal is as follows: in a small bowl, combine the garlic powder, paprika, and black pepper.

Place the chicken on a baking tray and entirely coat with the spice mixture. Transfer the chicken in the oven and bake for 60 minutes at 350 degrees F. Once chicken is juicy, chop the parts and serve on a plate.

#103 2-Cheese Baked Chicken Breasts

You will need 1/2 cup Parmesan cheese, 6 pieces chicken breast, 1/2 cup cheddar cheese, and 1/2 cup ranch dressing.

On a plate, arrange the chicken breasts in a row and pour randy dressing. In a bowl, combine the two cheeses. Transfer the chicken breasts in a baking dish; coat with the 2 cheeses. Bake for 20 to 30 minutes at 350 degrees F. Once done, serve on a plate and garnish with steamed veggies of your choice.

#104 Grilled Chicken and Bacon Kabobs in Spicy BBQ

You will need 2 chipotle peppers in adobo sauce, 8 bacon strips, 1/4 cup apple butter, 6 pieces chicken breasts, and 1 cup BBQ sauce.

Use steel skewers to thread the bacon and chicken; season with a dash of pepper. Meanwhile, in a blender, add the chipotle, apple butter and BBW sauce; blend until smooth. While grilling the chicken and bacon, brush the spicy BBQ sauce. Once done, serve while hot.

#105 Celery and Yellow Onion Citrus Chicken

1 chopped green bell pepper, 3 lbs. chicken, 3 lemons, 1/2 yellow onions, 2 celery stalks, 1/2 tbsp. thyme, 2 chopped carrots, 2 garlic cloves, 1 tbsp. rosemary, 2 bay leaves, and 1 cup chicken broth.

Stuff the chicken with one lemon and place in a crockpot. Cover chicken with seasonings and vegetables; pour the broth and lemon juice over the chicken. Cook the chicken for 8 hours over low heat. Serve on a plate and enjoy!

#106 Chicken Strips with Tomatoes and Zucchini

For this delicious and light meal, you need 2 turkey breasts. 1/4 cup black olives, 1/2 teaspoon oregano leaves, ½ cup green bell pepper, 1 tablespoon light butter, ½ cup yellow bell pepper, 2 zucchinis, and ½ cup red bell pepper.

For starters, in a bowl, add the chicken breast and sprinkle it with pepper. Add the zucchini slices and assorted bell peppers in foil. Top the vegetable mixture with the chicken, oregano, butter, tomato sauce and olives. Bake for 30 minutes at 250 degrees F.

#107 Chicken Strips with Tomatoes and Asparagus

This is variation #1. Replace zucchini with 2 asparagus bunches.

#108 Chicken Strips with Tomatoes and Parsnips

This is variation #2. Replace zucchini with 2 parsnips.

#109 Chicken Strips with Tomatoes and Celery

This is variation #3. Replace zucchini with 2 celery stalks.

#110 Chicken Strips with Tomatoes and Kale

This is variation #4. Replace zucchini with 1 lb. kale leaves.

#111 Chicken Strips with Tomatoes and Arugula

This is variation #5. Replace zucchini with 1 lb. arugula leaves.

#112 Chicken Salad in Whole Wheat Bagel Sandwiches

2 tbsp. lemon juice, 1 teaspoon dill seed, 1 onion, 2 chicken breasts, 2 tbsp. fresh parsley, 2 cups plain yogurt, 1 cup celery, and pepper to taste.

In a saucepan, add chicken, onions, celery stalks and water. Simmer the first 3 ingredients for 20 minutes and drain the water. Remove the chicken from pan, chop and set aside. In a medium bowl, add the plain yogurt, pepper, dill, lemon juice, celery and chicken. Fold the egg salad mixture and refrigerate for 30 minutes before serving on whole wheat bagels.

#113 Thyme and Mustard Grilled Chicken

1/2 teaspoon dried thyme, 4 pieces chicken breast halves, 1/4 cup cider vinegar, 1/2 teaspoon cayenne pepper, 1 and 1/4 teaspoons onion powder, 4 tablespoon salad oil, 1 medium carrot, 1/4 teaspoon dry mustard, 1 small red sweet pepper, 1/2 teaspoon black pepper, 1/4 teaspoon garlic powder, 1 green onion, and 6 cups mixed salad greens.

Set your grill temperature to 170 degrees F. Combine the onion powder, salad oil, cayenne pepper and pepper. Brush the oil mixture on the chicken and grill for 15 minutes until cooked through. Combine the mixed salad greens, green onion, red sweet pepper, and carrots in a large salad bowl. Add the chicken and pour the dressing before serving.

#114 Poached Chicken Thighs in Garlic and Radish

You will need the following ingredients to create this low-carb dish. Ghee (for frying), 2 and ½ lbs. chicken thighs, 7 pieces of radish (washed and halved), 3 pieces of carrots (sliced), 1 tablespoon of butter, 1 leek (washed and sliced into halves), 4 cloves garlic (halved and minced), and pepper to taste.

For the directions, season the chicken thighs with pepper and place them in a pot. Fill the pot with water and bring it to a boil. Add the carrots, garlic and leeks to the pot and simmer for 60 minutes. In a skillet, add coconut oil, garlic and radish. Transfer the cooked chicken to a plate and shred. Serve on a plate and top with radish and garlic.

#115 Poached Chicken Thighs in Garlic and Parsnips

This is variation #3. Replace radish with 7 pieces of parsnips.

#116 Chicken Whole-Wheat Fajitas with Fresh Salsa

1 small green sweet pepper, 12 ounces chicken breast strips, 1/3 cup cheddar cheese (reduced-fat), 1/4 teaspoon garlic powder, 2 10-inch whole wheat tortillas, 2 tablespoons ranch salad dressing (reduced-calorie), cooking spray, 1/2 teaspoon chili powder, and 1/2 cup fresh salsa.

Preheat your oven to 350 degrees F. In a medium-sized skillet, spray cooking oil and add the chicken strips, garlic powder and chili powder. Cook the ingredients for about 6 minutes to remove the rawness of the chicken and to soften the sweet peppers. Once done, transfer the pepper and chicken to a plate and set aside. Line the tortillas in the oven for 10 minutes until it blisters and heats up. Remove when done and transfer to a plate. Get the chicken and red green peppers, sprinkle a handful of cheddar cheese and place it on the warm tortilla. Wrap the tortilla in a foil and place it back in the oven.

#117 Cucumber and Chicken Pita Gyro

This recipe is good for those who love Mediterranean gyros. All you need is 1/2 pound chicken breasts, 1/2 cup cucumber, 1/2 teaspoon ground mustard, 2 tablespoons olive oil, 1/4 cup lemon juice, 1/4 teaspoon dill weeds, 1 garlic clove, 1/2 teaspoon dried oregano, 1/3 cup plain yogurt, 1/2 small red onion, and 2 whole pita breads.

To prepare this recipe, combine the olive oil, lemon juice, garlic, oregano and mustard in a zip-lock bag. Add the chicken and seal the zip-lock bag; refrigerate for an hour. Meanwhile, combine the yogurt, cucumber, garlic and dill weeds; refrigerate for 15 minutes. After an hour, remove the chicken from the bag and transfer to a large skillet. Cook the chicken for 8 minutes and when done, add them into the pita pockets. Top the chicken gyros with onions and yogurt mixture and serve.

#118 Chicken Gyro with Asparagus and Dill

Here is variation #1. Replace ½ cup cucumber with 1 bunch of asparagus.

#119 Chicken Gyro with Arugula and Dill

Here is variation #2. Replace ½ cup cucumber with 1 ½ cup chopped arugula leaves.

#120 Apple-Chicken Pita with Nutmeg and Garlic

To prepare a filling lunch, prepare these ingredients: 1 lb. chicken breast, 2 apples, 1 tablespoon olive oil, 2 large pitas, 2 garlic cloves, 2 cups onions, 1 tablespoon unsalted butter, 1/2 teaspoon cinnamon, 1/2 teaspoon ground nutmeg, and 1/2 teaspoon black pepper (freshly ground).

Cook the meal by starting sautéing chopped chicken breasts with olive oil in a pan; add nutmeg, pepper, cinnamon and salt. Remove the chicken and add unsalted butter; sauté the onions, garlic and apples for 6 minutes. Return the chicken and heat for 2 minutes. In a microwavable dish, add the pita and warm them in the microwave. Spread the chicken mixture and roll it. Serve on a plate and enjoy!

#121 Tropical Rings of Bacon and Chicken

1 bag of pre-washed romaine lettuce, ½ tbsp. fat-free mayonnaise, 2 bacon slices, 1 chicken breast, 1 tomato, 2 pineapple rings, and pepper to taste.

In a skillet, cook the bacon to a crisp; set the bacon fat aside. In the same skillet, pour bacon fat and cook the chicken for 5 minutes per side. Take the cooked chicken breasts and soak them in pineapple juice. Leave the chicken to soak up the juices for approximately four minutes. Get a large leaf of one lettuce and put a dollop of mayonnaise over it. Add the grilled pineapple slices, chicken, bacon and tomato. Roll the lettuce or make it like a taco and serve.

#122 Chicken Breast with Smokey Cherries and Apples

Prepare 4 chicken breasts and make the marinade. you need 1 can concentrated Cherry-Apple mix, 1/2 cup of vinegar, and 1 tsp. ground cinnamon. For the stuffing, you will need1 bag of cherries, 1 large apple, 1 cup chopped walnuts, and 1 bag fresh cranberries.

In a microwavable bowl, mix ingredients for the marinade. Place in the microwave oven for 20 seconds and allow it cool for a bit before pouring in a zip lock bag. Transfer the chicken breasts from the plate to the bag and seal it. Leave the chicken to marinade for as much as 8 hours. Set the smoker to 250 degrees F and directly set the chicken along the rack. Once the chicken is done, serve on a plate with almond slivers on the top.

#123 Chicken and Glazed Berries

This is variation #1. Replace the cherries and apples with 1 can concentrate raspberries.

#124 Smoked Cranberry-Chicken with Walnuts

This is variation #2. Replace the cherries and apples 1 can concentrate cranberry. Replace almond slivers with walnuts.

#125 Stuffed Chicken Breasts with Strawberry-Almond Filling

1 handful spinach, 1/2 cup balsamic vinegar, 16 ounces strawberries, 1 red onion, 1/2 cup of olive oil, 1 cup almonds, 1/4 cup of lemon juice, coconut oil for frying), and a dash of cinnamon.

In a pan, add the coconut oil, red onion and almond shavings. Wait until the onions have caramelized before adding the strawberries. Stir in the spinach and continue cooking for about 2 minutes. In a zip lock bag, mix olive oil, lemon juice, vinegar, olive oil. Include the chicken and marinate for 30 minutes in the refrigerator. Take the chicken out and pound it with a mallet. Once they are in fillet form, spoon in the assortment of strawberry and almonds. Roll the chicken fillet and line them in the sauté pan. Sprinkle a dash of cinnamon and place it in the oven. After baking the chicken, transfer the pan to a stove to sear the chicken for 25 minutes just in time before serving.

#126 Chicken with Rosemary and Peaches

2 tbsp. olive oil, 3 peaches, 1 sweet onion (thinly chopped), ¼ tsp. ground pepper, 4 rosemary sprigs, ¼ cup of raw honey, ¼ cup of balsamic vinegar, and 10 pieces chicken thighs.

Use a sauté pan and bring the olive oil to a medium high heat; sauté the rosemary, pepper, salt and onion for 5 minutes. Add the peaches and onion and sauté for another five minutes until the onions have turned translucent. Simmer the ingredients while adding balsamic vinegar and raw honey. Place the thighs in a baking dish and bake for 1 hour and a half at 375 degrees F. Place the liquid in a saucepan and boil for 3 minutes. Once the sauce thickens once more, pour along the chicken thighs and serve.

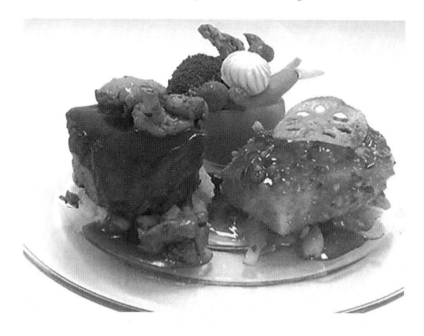

Category: Beef, Recipe #127-143

#127 Lean Ham with Toasts and Salsa

Prepare 2 thick slices of hard bread, 1 slice of lean ham, 1 egg, 4 tbsp. non-fat milk, 3 tbsp. unsalted butter, 1 tbsp. olive oil, and 1 jar of tomato salsa (store-bought).

To make it, spread butter on a slice of bread and add a slice of ham; cover with another bread. In a deep bowl, whisk an egg and pour milk; season with pepper. Dip the sandwich in the egg mixture and transfer to a pan. In a pan, add butter and fry the sandwich for about 2 minutes or until it turns golden brown. Serve on a plate and add a small bowl of tomato salsa for dipping.

#128 Baked Beef Sausage Ciabatta

You need 8 ounces Ciabatta bread, 1 cup sharp cheddar cheese (reduced fat), 1/2 cup green onions, 1 lb. beef breakfast sausage, 1 and 1/4 cups fat-free milk, cooking spray, 2 tablespoons fresh parsley, and 2 large eggs.

To make it, line the Ciabatta bread cubes in one layer and bake in the oven for 8 minutes at 400 degrees F. When the Ciabatta turns golden brown, remove from it from the oven. In a pan, coat cooking spray and add the sausages. Add beaten eggs, cheese, and milk. Combine the egg mixture with the bread mixture; set aside. Refrigerate for 1 hour. Bake the casserole for 50 minutes at 400 degrees F. Once it is ready, remove and serve.

#129 Grilled Bruschetta with Portobello, Ham and Cheese

To make this, get 2 slices lean beef ham, 2 slices hard country bread, 4 large Portobello mushrooms, 2 teaspoons olive oil (extra-virgin), 2 tablespoons Parmesan cheese, 1 garlic clove and cooking spray.

Once you are ready, place the mushrooms on the grill rack and grill for 5 minutes until lightly browned; transfer to a plate. Cut the bread into halves and grill for 1 minute. Halfway through grilling, rub the bread with a clove of garlic and drizzle olive oil. Use a small pan to sauté the mushrooms in olive oil. Once the mushrooms soften, prepare the grilled bruschetta. Top each bruschetta with ham, parmesan cheese, and mushrooms.

#130 Garlicky Ricotta Bacon and Mini Peppers

6 ounces soft goat cheese, 1 teaspoon garlic powder, 15 sweet mini peppers, 15 bacon strips, 1/2 cup ricotta cheese, and pepper (to taste).

Set oven to broil and line a baking sheet with foil; set aside. In a small bowl, add the ricotta, seasonings and goat cheese. Pipe in the cheese mixture into the halved peppers; wrap in bacon. Broil the arranged peppers for about 56 minutes until it turns nicely brown before serving on a plate.

#131 Chili in Pinto Beans and Beef

large onion, 1 large bell pepper, 2 lb. ground beef, 2 cans diced tomatoes, 3 jalapeno peppers, 1/2 cup chili powder, 1 teaspoon crushed red pepper flakes, 3 cans pinto beans, 4 cans tomato sauce, 1 teaspoon ground black pepper, and 1/4 teaspoon garlic powder.

In a large pot, add the onion, bell pepper and ground beef; cook for 10 minutes. Stir in the rest of the ingredients; bring ground beef mixture to a rolling boil. Simmer the chili for 30 minutes and serve in bowls.

#132 Garlic-Radish Beef Tenderloin Tips

1 lb. tenderloin steak, ground black pepper (to taste), 2 pieces radish, 1 and ½ tablespoons oil, 2 cloves garlic, 2 tablespoons sake, and scallions (for garnishing).

In a bowl, add the grated radish, scallions and garlic. On a chopping board, trim off excess fat from the tenderloin tips; season it with pepper. In a frying pan, add oil and sauté the garlic until lightly brown. Transfer the garlic on paper towels to drain excess oil; retain garlic oil in the pan. Cook the steak in the pan until it turns brown; flip to continue cooking the other side. Pour sake and shake pan to distribute evenly. Place the tenderloin tips on a plate; garnish with grated radish, crunchy garlic and scallions.

#133 Beef Tenderloin Tips with Garlic and Parsnips

This is variation #1. Replace radish with 2 pieces of parsnips.

#134 Spicy Beef with Zucchini and Mushrooms Skillet

1 1/3 pound beef, 1 cup chopped celery, 1 tablespoon chopped garlic, 2 cups chopped onions, 5 ounces sliced mushrooms, ground pepper (to taste), 2 cups chopped zucchini, and 1 tablespoon olive oil.

In a medium-sized pot, add celery, garlic and onions; cook until onions turn translucent. Add in the mushrooms, beef, zucchini and pepper; cook for 15 minutes. Season mushroom mixture with ground pepper and red pepper flakes; serve in a big plate and enjoy.

#135 Spicy Beef with Radish and Mushrooms Skillet

Here is variation #1. Replace zucchini with 2 cups chopped radish.

#136 Spicy Beef with Parsnip-Mushrooms Skillet

Here is a variation #2. Replace zucchini with 2 cups chopped parsnips.

#137 Moroccan Beef Burger with a Tower of Onions

1 sweet onion (large), 1 tablespoon olive oil (for sautéing), 3 onions, 1 tablespoon coconut oil, pepper to taste, 1 lb. ground beef, and1 tablespoon Cajun seasoning . In a skillet, simmer onions in olive oil for 30 minutes.

Season caramelized onions with a dash of pepper. Prepare the burgers by mixing the season and meat. Add coconut oil on a skillet and cook the meat for 5 minutes. Serve the beef with caramelized onions.

#138 Tomato-Beef Hamburger Macaroni Skillet

1 and 1/2 pounds ground beef, 2 cans tomato soup, 2 cups elbow macaroni (uncooked), 2 cups frozen mixed vegetables, 2 cups water, 2 teaspoons garlic powder, 1 teaspoon dried basil, and 1/2 teaspoon dried oregano.

In a large skillet, cook the ground beef; drain. Add the tomato soup together with macaroni, basil, garlic powder, mixed vegetables, water, and oregano; bring to a rolling boil. After the first boil, reduce the heat and simmer for 20 minutes or until macaroni is tender.

#139 Summer BBQ Beef Burger

1 can of pineapple rings, 1 beef burger, 8 slices cheddar cheese (fat-free), 8 hamburger buns, 1 head of lettuce, 1 tomato, 1 plain yogurt, and 1 bottle BBQ sauce.

In a pan, coat with cooking spray and add a pineapple ring; cook until caramelized; set aside. Top the burger with BBQ sauce, add cheese; microwave for 30 seconds. Once the cheese melts, add the pineapple ring on top and cover the bread. Top with tomato and romaine lettuce.

#140 Baked Beef Meatballs in a Classic Mustard Dip

1 package cheddar cheese, vegetable oil (to coat cookie sheet), 1 lb. beef sausage, 1 bottle Dijon mustard, 2 cups all-purpose flour, and fresh Cilantro leaves (for garnishing).

In a mixing bowl, add the all-purpose flour baking mix, water and cheese. In a cookie sheet, line aluminum foil and coat it with vegetable oil. After making the dough, roll it to a ball and put the sliced sausages in the middle and pop it in the oven for 12 minutes at 400 degrees F. When the sausage roll is done, remove from the cookie sheet and drain excess oil on a paper towel. Serve with a mustard dip and garnish with cilantro.

#141 Polish Spicy Sausage with Green Lentil and Carrots

To make this hearty soup, you will need 3 cans of chicken broth, 1 tbsp. dried thyme, 2 large garlic cloves, 1 tbsp. kosher salt, 1 pound Polish sausage, 1 lb. green lentils, , 4 cups leeks, 1 1/2 tsp. freshly ground black pepper, 1/4 cup olive oil, 1/4 cup tomato paste, 1 tsp. ground cumin, 4 cups yellow onions (minced) Parmesan cheese (for topping), 2 tbsp. red wine vinegar, 8 celery stalks, and 6 carrots.

In a pot, bring water to a rolling boil and add the lentils; drain and set aside. In a pot, sauté leeks, onions, salt, garlic, thyme, cumin and pepper for 20 minutes. Once the vegetables are tender, add carrots and celery; cook for 10 minutes then remove from the pot. Use the same pot and boil tomato paste, chicken stock and lentils. Simmer for an hour before adding the red wine and Polish sausages. To serve, ladle in bowls and top with grated Parmesan cheese.

#142 Beef Tenderloins in Sautéed Olive and Zucchini

This recipe will require you 1 small diced onion, 3 minced garlic cloves, 2 teaspoons garlic powder, 1/2 lb. beef tenderloin strips,1 teaspoon ground allspice, 1 large diced zucchini, 1 tablespoon dried oregano 1 can diced tomatoes, 1/2 cup green olives, and pepper to taste.

You will need a large skillet. Heat the lamb until fat comes out; add garlic, onions and all the spices. In the same skillet, add the olives and zucchini with liquid that came from the olives. Add tomatoes then reduce heat. Simmer for 20 minutes; season with pepper.

#143 Beef Tenderloins in Olives and Asparagus

Here is variation #1. Replace zucchini with 2 bunches of asparagus.

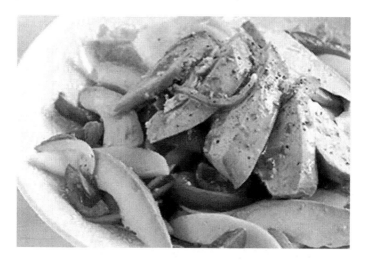

Category: Turkey, Recipes #144-150

#144 Turkey with Rosemary and Garlic

To make the recipe, you need 3 cloves garlic, 2 lb. turkey chunks, 1/4 cup fresh lemon juice, 1 tablespoon black peppercorns, 2 tablespoons fresh rosemary, and 2 tablespoons olive oil.

To prepare, you need to preheat your grill and grease the pan with cooking spray. In a medium-sized bowl, add the garlic, turkey chunks, lemon juice, peppercorns and rosemary; refrigerate for 1 hour. Remove the turkey from marinade. In a pan, cook the turkey for about 4 minutes; add the remaining lemon juice. Serve on a plate and garnish with rosemary leaves.

#145 Smoked Turkey with Mango-Arugula Salad

1/4 cup fresh cilantro, 4 cups smoked turkey, lime vinaigrette (store-bought), 4 cups salad greens, and 2 medium diced mangoes.

On a chopping board, peel and slice the ripe mangoes by about 1/8 of an inch. Prepare a bowl and add chopped turkey, cilantro; toss in the arugula. Serve on a plate and drizzle lime vinaigrette on top.

#146 Turkey Strips with Tomatoes and Zucchini

For this delicious and light meal, you need 2 turkey breasts. 1/4 cup black olives, 1/2 teaspoon oregano leaves, ½ cup green bell pepper, 1 tablespoon light butter, ½ cup yellow bell pepper, 2 zucchinis, and ½ cup red bell pepper.

For starters, in a bowl, add the chicken breast and sprinkle it with pepper. Add the zucchini slices and assorted bell peppers in foil. Top the vegetable mixture with the chicken, oregano, butter, tomato sauce and olives. Bake for 30 minutes at 250 degrees F.

#147 Turkey Strips with Tomatoes and Asparagus

Here is variation #1. Replace zucchini with 2 bunches of asparagus.

#148 Turkey Strips with Tomatoes and Radish

Here is variation #2. Replace 2 cups zucchini with 2 cups chopped radish.

#149 Turkey Strips with Tomatoes and Celery

Here is variation #3. Replace zucchini with 2 cups chopped celery stalks.

#150 Turkey Strips with Tomatoes and Parsnips

Here is variation #4. Replace zucchini with 2 cups chopped parsnips.

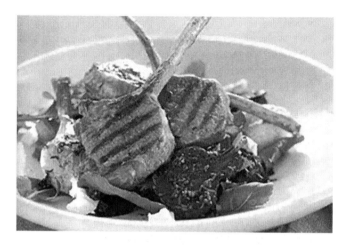

Category: Lamb, Recipes #151-158

#151 Lamb Salad with Cranberries and Almonds

For this recipe, you will need 4 tablespoons light cream cheese, 1 cup fat-free mayonnaise, 2 teaspoons curry powder; 6 cups pre-cooked lamb cubes, 2/3 cup dried cranberries, and 1 cup almonds.

In a large bowl, add cream cheese, and curry powder. Whisk the ingredients and mix cranberries and lamb. Transfer the mixture in a plastic round cake pan and refrigerate for 2 hours. Toss the salad and garnish with chopped almonds and cranberries on top.

#152 Tropical Ring BBQ Lamb Burger

1 can of pineapple rings, 1 lamb burger, 8 slices cheddar cheese (fat-free), 8 hamburger buns, 1 head of lettuce, 1 tomato, 1 plain yogurt, and 1 bottle BBQ sauce.

In a pan, coat with cooking spray and add a pineapple ring; cook until caramelized; set aside. Top the burger with BBQ sauce, add cheese; microwave for 30 seconds. Once the cheese melts, add the pineapple ring on top and cover bread. Top with a tomato and romaine lettuce.

#153 Mediterranean Lamburgini

1 lb. ground lamb, 1 onion, 2 garlic cloves, 1 tbsp. dried dill, and 1/2 teaspoon black pepper.

Mix the ingredients in a large bowl until everything is well combined. Shape the ground lamb into burgers. Fry them in a pan and cook for 5 minutes per side. Fill wheat bread burgers with the lamburgini, romaine lettuce and Dijon mustard.

#154 Lamb Gyros in Rosemary and Oregano

3 lbs. lamb, 1 package pita bread, 2 teaspoons ground dried rosemary, 2 tablespoons olive oil, pepper (for seasoning), 1 tablespoon minced garlic, 1 1/2 tablespoons ground cumin, 1 tablespoon red wine vinegar, and 1 tablespoon dried oregano.

In a large ceramic bowl, add the cumin, garlic, rosemary, red wine vinegar, venison strips, oregano, and pepper; toss to coat the meat. Cover the ceramic bowl and refrigerate the marinade for about 2 hours. Cook lamb strips in a large skillet for about 8 minutes until golden brown.

#155 Pan-Seared Lamb in Zucchini and Olives

1 small diced onion, 3 minced garlic cloves, 2 teaspoons garlic powder, 1 lb. ground lamb, 1 teaspoon ground allspice, 1 tablespoon dried oregano, 1 large diced zucchini, 1 can diced tomatoes, 1/2 cup pitted olives, and pepper to taste.

In a large skillet, heat the lamb until fat comes out; add garlic, onions and all the spices. In the same skillet, add the olives and zucchini with liquid that came from the olives. Add tomatoes; simmer for 20 minutes. Once done, serve on a plate and sprinkle pepper to taste.

#156 Pan-Seared Lamb in Parsnips and Olives

Here is variation #1. Replace zucchini with 2 cups chopped parsnips.

#157 Pan-Seared Lamb Roast with Lemon Juice and Spices

To make this recipe, you will need 4 legs of lamb, 1 tsp. black pepper, 2 tbsp. fresh mint (finely chopped), 2 tbsp. lemon juice, 2 tbsp. olive oil, 3 garlic cloves, 2 tsp. paprika, 1 tsp. ground cumin, and a pinch of cayenne powder.

In a small bowl, combine all the ingredients and rub on the lamb. In pressure cooker, set the temperature high for 40 minutes; place 4 legs of lamb together with a cup of water for steaming. Transfer the breaded leg of lamb on a roasting pan; sear until golden brown.

#158 Grilled Lamb Skewers in Minty Yogurt Dip

To make this recipe, you will need 1 tbsp. mint sauce (store-bought), 13 oz. lean lamb, 1 container plain yogurt, 14 oz. couscous, ground black pepper (to taste), 2 small onions, 1 green bell pepper, 1 garlic clove, 8 lemon wedges, 2 tbsp. chopped mint, and 8 pieces wooden bamboo skewers.

Directions: in a medium-sized bowl, combine the mint sauce, mint, garlic and lamb. Cover lamb with the mint sauce mixture; refrigerate for 10 minutes. In a large bowl, add the couscous and pour boiling water; allow rice to absorb water before seasoning it with pepper. Thread the onion and lemon wedges. Heat a grill and cook until grill marks appear on the lamb. Serve the kebabs with the cooked couscous, and sour cream.

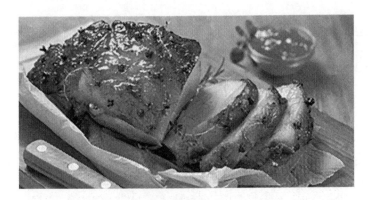

Category: Pork, Recipes #159-160

#159 Pork Barbecue with Sautéed Onions and Garlic

1 teaspoon garlic (chopped), 1 cup onions (chopped, 1 tablespoon olive oil, 4 pork chops, 1 cup barbecue sauce (bottled), 1/4 teaspoon freshly ground black pepper, and 1/2 cup water.

In a medium-sized skillet, sauté the garlic and onions in olive oil; retain the drippings and add the chops. Remove the chops; add the salt, BBQ sauce, pepper and water. Transfer the chops back, simmer for 45 minutes. Serve in a plate and enjoy!

#160 Dockside BBQ Pork Baguette Sandwiches

1 bottle barbeque sauce, 1 can beef broth, French bread or baguette, and 3 pounds pork ribs. Preheat your oven to 350 degrees F.

Prepare a slow cooker, add the beef broth together with pork ribs and cook on high heat for about four hours. Once the meat is done, shred and transfer it to an iron skillet. Bake the pork ribs for about 30 minutes and set aside to cool. Slice one whole baguette in half and slice it horizontally to open the middle. In a small bowl, add the boneless pork ribs and toss to coat with barbecue sauce. Add the pork ribs in the sliced bread and serve with potato chips or fries.

Chapter 3

Mediterranean Low-Carb Dinner Recipes

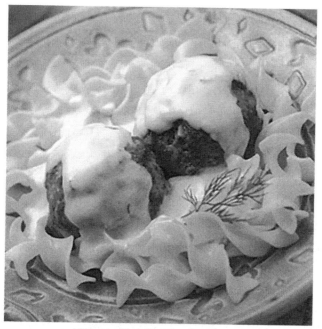

Photo Credit: landolakes

A typical Mediterranean dinner is light and easy to prepare. Lunch happens to be the second heaviest meal. In this chapter, get to learn quick pasta recipes, salad and soup. Some meals are considered part of the comfort food category since it has creams and rich flavors. That is why the chosen recipes are prepared in olive oil and vinegar.

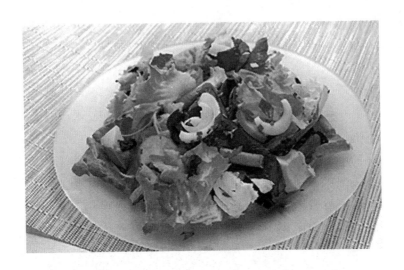

Category: Salad, Recipes #161-214

#161 Meat lover's Sandwich with Olive Salad

1/2 cup olive oil, 1 tablespoon capers, 3 finely minced cloves garlic, 1/3 cup parsley (finely chopped, 1 teaspoon oregano, 1 cup green olives, 1 mashed fillet of anchovy, 1 cup black olives, 1/4 teaspoon black pepper, and 1/4 cup chopped pimiento.

In a large bowl, mix all the ingredients for the olive salad and marinate them for 1 hour. Slice the bread in half and add salami, ham and provolone cheese. Add the olive salad mixture on the bread. Serve on a plate and enjoy!

#162 Sautéed Beef in Tomatoes and Avocado Salad

8 cups Romaine Lettuce, 1 chopped green bell pepper, ¼ wedged lime, 1 tsp. onion powder, 1 tsp. garlic powder, 1 tbsp. chili powder, 1 avocado, 1 lb. lean ground beef, 1 chopped tomato, and 1 cup salsa.

Season the ground beef with all the spices and cook it until it is halfway down. Chop the vegetables, put the beef on a plate and put salsa on top. Before serving, squeeze lime juice for added flavor.

#163 Beef Salad with Cranberries and Almonds

For this recipe, you will need 4 tablespoons light cream cheese, 1 cup fat-free mayonnaise, 2 teaspoons curry powder; 6 cups pre-cooked beef chunks, 2/3 cup dried cranberries, and 1 cup almonds. In a large bowl, add cream cheese, and curry powder.

Whisk the ingredients and mix cranberries and beef. Transfer the mixture in a plastic round cake pan and refrigerate for 2 hours. Toss the salad and garnish with chopped almonds and cranberries on top.

#164 Madagascar Lentils, Collard Greens, and Brown Rice

2 teaspoons extra-virgin olive oil, 1 tomato, 1/2 onions, ¼ teaspoon fresh ginger root, 1/2 bunch collard greens, 3 cups water, 2 cups brown rice, and black pepper (to taste).

In a large skillet, sauté onions, ginger and tomatoes in olive oil; cook for about 3 minutes until it turns soft. Stir in the chopped collard greens into the ginger and tomato mixture; cook until vegetables are done. Transfer the skillet contents into a slow cooker, add rice and water. Cook for 4 hours until rice is done.

#165 Chicken and Tomato-Zucchini Salad

To prepare this mouthwatering lunch, you need 2 chicken breasts, 2 tablespoons tomato sauce, 1/4 cup black olives, 1/2 teaspoon oregano leaves, ½ cup green bell pepper, 1 tablespoon light butter ,½ cup yellow bell pepper, 2 medium zucchini, and ½ cup red bell pepper.

Directions: In a bowl, add the chicken breast, zucchini slices and assorted bell peppers; wrap in a fall. Top the vegetable mixture with chicken, oregano, butter, tomato sauce and olives. Bake for 30 minutes at 250 degrees F. Unwrap the foil and serve immediately.

#166 Chicken and Tomato-Parsnip Salad

Here is variation #1. Replace 2 zucchinis with 2 parsnips.

#167 Chicken and Tomato-Cucumber Salad

Here is variation #2. Replace 2 zucchinis with 2 cucumbers.

#168 Chicken and Tomato-Asparagus Salad

Here is variation #2. Replace 2 zucchinis with 2 asparagus bunch.

#169 Tuna and Black Olives Salad in Vinegar

A healthy lunch includes this vegetable salad. You will need 2 tbsp. white wine vinegar, 1/2 cup black olives, 1/4 cup of olive oil, 1 cabbage (cut into strips), 1 can tuna in oil, 2 cups fresh curly parsley, and 1/2 red onion.

Here is the direction: in a salad bowl, add pepper, salt, and white wine vinegar; whisk to emulsify. Add the rest of the ingredients and toss to combine. Refrigerate for 30 minutes and serve chilled.

#170 Tuna-Spinach Salad with Walnuts

Spinach leaves (a handful), 1 package Albacore tuna (in water), 1 large diced carrot

¼ cup raisins, 1 tomato, and chopped walnuts (for topping).

Add the tomato slices and carrots on top of the spinach. Top with tuna, walnuts and raisins. Serve and enjoy the salad.

#171 Salmon-Spinach Salad with Walnuts

Here is variation #1. Replace with 500 g. salmon.

#172 Salmon-Asparagus Salad with Walnuts

Here is variation #2. Replace with 2 asparagus bunches.

#173 Salmon-Arugula Salad with Walnuts

Here is variation #3. Replace with 2 Arugula bunches.

#174 Mahi Mahi-Spinach Salad with Walnuts

Here is variation #4. Replace with 500 g. Mahi Mahi.

#175 Mahi Mahi-Asparagus Salad with Walnuts

Here is variation #5. Replace with 2 asparagus bunches.

#176 Mahi Mahi-Arugula Salad with Walnuts

Here is variation #6. Replace with 2 Arugula bunches.

#177 Cod-Spinach Salad with Walnuts

Here is variation #7. Replace with 500 g. Cod fillet.

#178 Cod-Asparagus Salad with Walnuts

Here is variation #8. Replace with 2 asparagus bunches.

#179 Cod-Arugula Salad with Walnuts

Here is variation #9. Replace with 2 Arugula bunches.

#180 Herring-Spinach Salad with Walnuts

Here is variation #10. Replace with 500 g. Herring fillet.

#181 Herring-Asparagus Salad with Walnuts

Here is variation #11. Replace with 2 asparagus bunches.

#182 Herring-Arugula Salad with Walnuts

Here is variation #12. Replace with 2 Arugula bunches.

#183 Radicchio-Pecan Salad in Balsamic Dressing

2 ounces toasted pecans, 225 ml extra virgin olive oil, 3 cloves garlic, 1 ounce dried cranberries, 3 bulbs fennel, 3 small heads radicchio, 2 tablespoons balsamic vinegar, 2 tablespoons red wine vinegar, and 3 bunches watercress.

In a small bowl, combine the red wine vinegar, garlic, cranberries, balsamic vinegar and salt. Slowly whisk in the olive oil to emulsify. In a large salad bowl, combine the radicchio, watercress, fennel and pecans. Pour the balsamic dressing over salad; toss well, top with shavings of non-dairy gorgonzola cheese and serve.

#184 Radicchio-Almond Salad in Balsamic Dressing

This is variation #1. Replace pecans with 2 ounces toasted almonds.

#185 Iceberg Lettuce-Pecan Salad in Balsamic Dressing

This is variation #2. Replace radicchio with 3 small heads iceberg lettuce.

#186 Iceberg Lettuce-Walnut Salad in Balsamic Dressing

This is variation #2. Replace pecan with 2 ounces toasted almonds.

#187 Mediterranean Tofu with Spinach-Red Cabbage Salad

2 tbsp. balsamic vinegar, 1 1/2 tsp. olive oil, 1 cup red cabbage, 1 tbsp. pine nuts, 3 oz. firm tofu, 1 cup chopped raw spinach, 1 oz. soft goat cheese, and 1/2 cup mandarin oranges (canned).

In a large bowl, add the red cabbage, pine nuts, tofu and the rest of the ingredients. Gently combine and serve on a plate. Top with pine nuts and a few pieces of raw spinach.

#188 Mediterranean Tofu with Arugula-Red Cabbage Salad

This is variation #1. Replace with arugula.

#189 Mediterranean Tofu with Kale-Red Cabbage Salad

This is variation #2. Replace with kale leaves.

#190 Mediterranean Tofu with Kale-Radicchio Salad

This is variation #3. Replace with radicchio.

#191 Broccoli, Carrots with Feta and Red Pepper Dip

To assemble this easy low-carb vegetable creamy dip, add 1 tsp. garlic, 1/2 cup roasted red peppers, 1/2 tsp. olive oil, 1/2 cup broccoli, 1/2 cup carrots, and 1/4 cup feta cheese.

Make the dip by blending the feta cheese, roasted red peppers, garlic, and olive oil in a food processor. As soon as the pepper mixture turns smooth, transfer it into a small serving bowl. Serve the dip with broccoli and carrots and enjoy!

#192 Asparagus, Carrots with Feta and Red Pepper Dip

This is variation #1. Replace with asparagus.

#193 Kale, Carrots with Feta and Red Pepper Dip

This is variation #2. Replace with kale.

#194 Cucumbers, Carrots with Feta and Red Pepper Dip

This is variation #3. Replace with cucumbers.

#195 Zucchini, Carrots with Feta and Red Pepper Dip

This is variation #4. Replace with zucchini.

#196 Cucumber and Tofu salad

Handful chopped fresh basil, 1 tin kidney bean, freshly ground black pepper to taste, 1 cucumber, 1 tomato, 1/2 red onion, 100g firm tofu, and 4 tablespoons salad dressing of choice.

In a large bowl, combine the cucumber, red onion, kidney beans, tofu, tomato and basil. Toss with balsamic dressing, season with salt and pepper. Serve on plate and enjoy with fresh shavings of a non-dairy cheese of choice.

#197 Asparagus and Tofu salad

This is variation #4. Replace with asparagus.

#198 Radish and Tofu salad

This is variation #4. Replace with radish.

#199 Parsnip and Tofu salad

This is variation #5. Replace with parsnip.

#200 Kale and Tofu salad

This is variation #6. Replace with kale.

#201 Celery and Tofu salad

This is variation #7. Replace with celery.

#202 Zucchini and Tofu salad

This is variation #8. Replace with zucchini.

#203 Red Cabbage and Tofu salad

Variation #9; replace with red cabbage.

#204 Romaine Lettuce and Tofu salad

Variation #9; replace with 1 head of lettuce.

#205 Butternut Pumpkin, Spinach Salad with Feta Cheese

1 butternut pumpkin, 300 grams baby spinach leaves, 1/4 cup olive oil (extra virgin), 1 tbsp. mustard (wholegrain), 2 tbsp. red wine vinegar, 200 grams feta cheese, and 3 red onions.

Preheat your barbecue grill and set the temperature to medium heat. Cut the butternut pumpkin to several slices, brush with olive oil and season with pepper. Grill the pumpkin slices until they become tender and put on a plate. On the same grill, add an onion and grill until translucent. In a large serving bowl, add the grilled pumpkin, grilled onion, feta cheese and spinach leaves. Prepare the dressing by combining the vinegar, olive oil and mustard then pour the contents into a jar. Toss the salad and serve with the vinaigrette dressing. Top with crumbled some feta cheese and serve.

#206 Butternut Pumpkin, Kale Salad with Feta Cheese

Variation #1; replace with 300 grams kale.

#207 Butternut Pumpkin, Asparagus Salad with Feta Cheese

Variation #2; replace with 4 asparagus bunches.

#208 Butternut Pumpkin, Romaine Lettuce Salad with Feta Cheese

Variation #3; replace with 1 head of lettuce.

#209 Chicken Breast Tomato-Cucumber Salad

2 chicken breasts, 2 tablespoons tomato sauce, 1/4 cup black olives, 1/2 teaspoon oregano leaves, ½ cup green bell pepper, 1 tablespoon unsalted butter, ½ cup red bell pepper, 2 medium cucumber, and ½ cup green bell pepper.

In a bowl, add the chicken breast and sprinkle it with pepper. In a foil wrap, add the cucumber slices and assorted bell peppers. Top the vegetable mixture with the chicken, oregano, unsalted butter, tomato sauce and olives. Wrap the foil and bake for 30 minutes at 250 degrees F.

#210 Chicken Breast Tomato-Parsnip Salad

This is variation #1. Replace 2 medium cucumbers with 2 parsnips.

#211 Chicken Breast Tomato-Asparagus Salad

This is variation #2. Replace with 2 asparagus bunches.

#212 Turkey Breast Tomato-Zucchini Salad

2 turkey breasts, 2 tablespoons tomato sauce, 1/4 cup black olives, 1/2 teaspoon oregano leaves, ½ cup green bell pepper, 1 tablespoon unsalted butter, ½ cup yellow bell pepper, 2 medium zucchini, and ½ cup red bell pepper.

In a bowl, add the turkey breast and sprinkle it with pepper. In a foil wrap, add the zucchini slices and assorted bell peppers. Top the vegetable mixture with the chicken, oregano, unsalted butter, tomato sauce and olives. Wrap the foil and bake for 30 minutes at 250 degrees F.

#213 Turkey Breast Tomato-Asparagus Salad

This is variation #1. Replace with 2 asparagus bunches.

#214 Turkey Breast Tomato-Parsnip Salad

This is variation #2. Replace with 2 Parsnips.

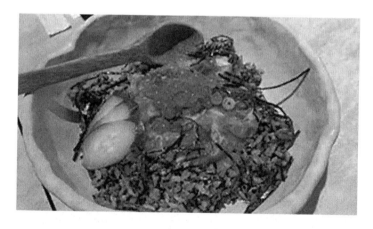

Category: Fish, Recipes #215-270

#215 Steamed Cream Dory Fillet in Chili-Tomato Quinoa

6 pieces steamed cream dory fillets, 1 can of tomatoes, 2 green chili peppers, 2 cups chicken broth, 1/4 cup chopped fresh cilantro, 1 cup quinoa, 1 packet taco seasoning mix, 1 jalapeno pepper, 1 small onion, 2 cloves garlic, and 1 tbsp. olive oil.

In a small pot, stir in chicken broth and quinoa and cook for 15 minutes. In a skillet, heat the olive oil and stir in the chopped jalapeno peppers, minced onions and garlic. Set the garlic aside before it turns golden brown. When the quinoa is done, return the garlic in the skillet and add the taco seasoning, diced tomatoes and chili; cook for 3 more minutes before turning the heat off. Serve the spicy quinoa on a plate and top with steamed fish fillet.

#126 Steamed Halibut Fillet in Chili-Tomato Quinoa

Variation #1; replace with halibut fillet.

#217 Steamed Herring Fillet in Chili-Tomato Quinoa

Variation #2; replace with herring fillet.

#218 Steamed Milkfish Fillet in Chili-Tomato Quinoa

Variation #3; replace with milkfish fillet.

#219 Steamed Cod Fillet in Chili-Tomato Quinoa

Variation #4; replace with milkfish fillet.

#220 Steamed Salmon Fillet in Chili-Tomato Quinoa

Variation #5; replace with salmon fillet.

#221 Red Snapper Fillet with Olives and Feta Cheese

6 pieces red snapper fillets, 2 tbsp. black olives, 2 tbsp. olive oil, 2 tbsp. low-fat feta cheese, ½ cup carrots, 1 large tomato, 1 clove garlic, ½ cup dry white wine, 1 medium onion, and ½ cup red pepper.

In a medium-sized skillet, sauté the carrots, red pepper, onions and garlic with olive oil; cook for 10 minutes. Add white wine and bring to a boil. Place the fish fillets in the same skillet and cook for about 5 minutes; add the olives and tomatoes. Cook the fillets for about 3 minutes top with cheese. Transfer to a serving plate; garnish with the skillet's juices and cooked vegetable. Serve with ½ cup of cooked brown rice.

#222 Halibut Fillet with Olives and Feta Cheese

Variation #1; replace with halibut fillet.

#223 Herring Fillet with Olives and Feta Cheese

Variation #2; replace with herring fillet.

#224 Milkfish Fillet with Olives and Feta Cheese

Variation #3; replace with milkfish fillet.

#225 Cod Fillet with Olives and Feta Cheese

Variation #4; replace with milkfish fillet.

#226 Salmon Fillet with Olives and Feta Cheese

Variation #5; replace with salmon fillet.

#227 Cod Fillet with Black and Green Olives Served with Feta

1 lb. cod fillet, 2 tbsp. black olives (chopped), 2 tbsp. green olives (chopped), 2 tbsp. olive oil, 2 tbsp. low-fat feta cheese, ½ cup carrots, 1 large tomato, 1 clove garlic , ½ cup dry white wine, 1 medium onion, and ½ cup red pepper.

In a medium-sized skillet, sauté the carrots, red pepper, onions and garlic with olive oil; cook for 10 minutes. Add white wine and bring to a boil. Place the cod fillet in the same skillet and cook for about 5 minutes; add the green and black olives and tomatoes. Cook the fillets for about 3 minutes top with cheese. Transfer to a serving plate; garnish with the skillet's juices and cooked vegetable. Serve with ½ cup of cooked brown rice.

#228 Red Snapper Fillet with Black and Green Olives Served with Feta

Variation #1; replace with halibut fillet.

#229 Halibut Fillet with Black and Green Olives Served with Feta

Variation #1; replace with halibut fillet.

#230 Herring Fillet with Black and Green Olives Served with Feta

Variation #2; replace with herring fillet.

#231 Milkfish Fillet with Black and Green Olives Served with Feta

Variation #3; replace with milkfish fillet.

#232 Salmon Fillet with Black and Green Olives Served with Feta

Variation #5; replace with salmon fillet.

#233 Olives and Haddock Fillets with Cherry Tomatoes

1 cup green olives, 2 tbsp. capers (pickled), 4 Haddock fish fillets, 1 clove garlic, 1 tbsp. Olive oil, 1 bunch fresh thyme, 500g cherry tomatoes, and pepper to taste.

In a heatproof bowl, add the cherry tomato halves and thyme. Place fillets on top of the cherry tomatoes. Add the olive oil, and pressed garlic; pressure cook for 5 minutes on high heat. Serve the fillets with cherry tomatoes and thyme.

#234 Salmon Fillets with Olive and Cherry Tomatoes

Variation #1; replace with salmon fillet.

#235 Milkfish Fillet with Olive and Cherry Tomatoes

Variation #2; replace with milkfish fillet.

#235 Herring Fillet with Olive and Cherry Tomatoes

Variation #3; replace with herring fillet.

#236 Halibut Fillet with Olive and Cherry Tomatoes

Variation #4; replace with halibut fillet.

#237 Red Snapper Fillet with Olive and Cherry Tomatoes

Variation #5; replace with red snapper fillet.

#238 Tuna Fillet with Olive and Cherry Tomatoes

Variation #6; replace with tuna fillet.

#239 Cod Fillet with Olive and Cherry Tomatoes

Variation #7; replace with cod fillet.

#240 Spicy Cod Fillet in Coconut Milk

½ lb. Cod fish fillet, 1 cup cherry tomatoes, 1 medium fresh ginger (julienned), 2 medium onions (julienned), 2 green chilies (julienned), 2 garlic cloves (pressed), 3 tbsp. curry powder, 2 cups coconut milk, 1 tbsp. lemon juice, and 6 bay leaves.

In a pressure cooker, add a teaspoon of cooking oil, curry leaves and fry for a minute. Add the garlic, onions, and ginger; sauté until onions turn translucent. Add the chilies, curry powder, tomatoes, coconut milk, salt, cod fish fillet and bay leaves; coat fish well. Bring the pressure cooker heat to a high and cook for 5 minutes with the lid closed. Once done, transfer the contents to a serving dish and add the lemon juice on top.

#241 Spicy Salmon Fillets in Coconut Milk

Variation #1; replace with salmon fillet.

#242 Spicy Milkfish Fillet in Coconut Milk

Variation #2; replace with milkfish fillet.

#243 Spicy Herring Fillet in Coconut Milk

Variation #3; replace with herring fillet.

#244 Spicy Halibut Fillet in Coconut Milk

Variation #4; replace with halibut fillet.

#245 Spicy Red Snapper Fillet in Coconut Milk

Variation #5; replace with red snapper fillet.

#246 Spicy Tuna Fillet with in Coconut Milk

Variation #6; replace with tuna fillet.

#247 Breaded Cream Dory with Lemon

1 tablespoon grated lemon zest, 1/2 cup dry bread crumbs, 4 tablespoons unsalted butter, 2 teaspoons chopped fresh thyme, pepper to taste, and 4 pieces cream dory fillet.

In a pan, add the cream dory fillets, sprinkle pepper, set aside. In a pan, heat lemon juice, unsalted butter and lime zest. Brush the cream dory fillets with the lemon mixture. Dip into a bowl of thyme and bread crumbs. Pop tray into an oven and bake for 15 minutes until golden brown.

#248 Breaded Halibut with Lemon

Variation #1; replace with halibut fillet.

#249 Breaded Tuna with Lemon

Variation #2; replace with tuna fillet.

#250 Breaded Cod with Lemon

Variation #3; replace with cod fillet.

#251 Breaded Herring with Lemon

Variation #4; replace with herring fillet.

#252 Breaded Mahi Mahi with Lemon

Variation #5; replace with Mahi Mahi fillet.

#253 Baked Cream Dory in Buttery Capers

To make this recipe, you will need 2 tbsp. olive oil, 2 tbsp. unsalted butter, 2 tbsp. lemon juice, 1 tbsp. fresh tarragon, 1 garlic clove, 5 pieces cream dory fillets, 1 tbsp. capers, and pepper to taste.

Bake this low carb dish by layering all 5 pieces of cream dory fillets on a tray; season with pepper. In a bowl, make the marinade by whisking the olive oil, garlic and lemon juice, Pour the marinade over the fillets and pop in the oven for 10 minutes at 450 degrees F. Meanwhile, in a bowl, add melted butter, heated capers and tarragon. Transfer baked fillets, spoon over the buttery capers and serve.

#254 Baked Halibut in Buttery Capers

Variation #1; replace with halibut fillet.

#255 Baked Tuna in Buttery Capers

Variation #2; replace with tuna fillet.

#256 Baked Cod in Buttery Capers

Variation #3; replace with cod fillet.

#257 Baked Herring in Buttery Capers

Variation #4; replace with herring fillet.

#258 Baked Mahi Mahi in Buttery Capers

Variation #5; replace with Mahi Mahi fillet.

#259 Baked Halibut Fillet in Lemon and Thyme

This is another take of the cream dory but if it is not in season, replace it with the meaty Halibut fillet instead. Serve with lemon wedges and enjoy!

#260 Baked Salmon in Lemon and Thyme

Variation #1; replace with salmon fillet.

#261 Baked Tuna in Lemon and Thyme

Variation #2; replace with tuna fillet.

#262 Baked Cod in Lemon and Thyme

Variation #3; replace with cod fillet.

#263 Baked Herring in Lemon and Thyme

Variation #4; replace with herring fillet.

#264 Baked Mahi Mahi in Lemon and Thyme

Variation #5; replace with Mahi Mahi fillet.

#265 Tilapia in Sour Cream Dip

This is a variation of the cream dory and halibut but if it is not in season, replace it with Tilapia fish instead. Add a dollop of sour cream and serve.

#266 Baked Halibut in Sour Cream Dip

Variation #1; replace with halibut fillet.

#267 Baked Tuna in Sour Cream Dip

Variation #2; replace with tuna fillet.

#268 Baked Cod in Sour Cream Dip

Variation #3; replace with cod fillet.

#269 Baked Herring in Sour Cream Dip

Variation #4; replace with herring fillet.

#270 Baked Mahi Mahi in Sour Cream Dip

Variation #5; replace with Mahi Mahi fillet.

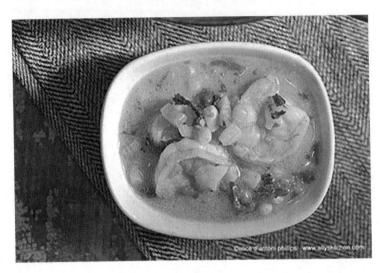

Category: Soup, Recipes #271-293

#271 Crawfish and Shrimp Stew

5 ounces medium shrimp, 1 clove garlic, 1 tablespoon plus 2 and 1/4 teaspoons vegetable oil, 5 ounces Crawfish tails, 1/2 medium onion, 1/2 small green bell pepper, 1/2 cup fish stock, 2 teaspoons hot sauce, 1/4 teaspoon ground cayenne pepper, 1 stalk celery, 1/4 teaspoon ground black pepper, 1 tablespoon

coconut flour, 5 fresh tomatoes, and 2 teaspoons seafood seasoning.

In a heavy skillet, add oil over medium heat. Prepare the roux by stirring in the flour with the oil for about 20 minutes. In the same skillet, add the garlic, onions and celery together with the bell peppers; sauté for 5 minutes to soften. Stir in the fish stock and chopped tomatoes; season with the seafood seasoning. Reduce the heat to low, simmer for 20 minutes; season with hot pepper sauce and cayenne pepper. Add the crawfish and shrimp then cook for 10 minutes.

#272 Salmon Fillets and Shrimp Stew

Variation #1; replace with salmon fillet.

#273 Milkfish Fillet and Shrimp Stew

Variation #2; replace with milkfish fillet.

#274 Herring Fillet and Shrimp Stew

Variation #3; replace with herring fillet.

#275 Halibut Fillet and Shrimp Stew

Variation #4; replace with halibut fillet.

#276 Red Snapper Fillet and Shrimp Stew

Variation #5; replace with red snapper fillet.

#277 Tuna Fillet and Shrimp Stew

Variation #6; replace with tuna fillet.

#278 Fillet with and Shrimp Stew

Variation #7; replace with cod fillet.

#279 Cod and Shrimp Stew in Coconut and Celery

This is a variation of the crawfish and shrimp stew. Use the cod fish; add 3 more celery stalks and season with kosher salt and pepper. Continue cooking it with the rest of the ingredients; serve while hot.

#280 Lamb and Apricots Stew

1 teaspoon dried thyme, 1 piece of white onion, 3 cloves of minced garlic, 2 cans of red kidney beans, 2 cups vegetable broth, 1 lb. shanks of lamb, 1 cup diced dried apricots, and pepper to taste).

Place the apricots, kidney beans, spices lamb shanks, broth and sliced onions in a crock pot, stir together to combine. Cook on high heat for about 6 hours. Once done, shred into flakes and mix to combine; serve in bowls.

#281 Beef and Apricots Stew

Variation #1; replace with 1 lb. beef.

#282 Chicken and Apricots Stew

Variation #2; replace with 1 whole chicken.

#283 Turkey and Apricots Stew

Variation #3; replace with 1 small turkey.

#284 Pumpkin- Sour Cream Soup with Whole Wheat Croutons

1 3/4 cup low-sodium vegetable broth, 2/3 cup pumpkin purée, 1 can diced tomatoes (reserve liquid), 2 cups nacho-blend cheese (shredded), 1 jalapeño, 1/4 cup light sour cream, 1/4 cup all-purpose flour, and parsley (for garnishing).

In a large pot, combine the vegetable broth, pumpkin puree and tomato liquid. Cook over medium heat for 3 minutes; remove from heat. Stir in nacho-blend cheese, sour cream, jalapeño and tomatoes. Bring soup to a boil; serve in individual bowls. Garnish with whole wheat croutons and parsley.

#285 Butternut Squash Soup with Whole Wheat Croutons

Variation #1; replace the pumpkin with butternut squash.

#286 Spicy Butternut Squash Soup with Apples and Carrots

To make this recipe, you will need 1 green apple (sliced and cored), 1 large butternut squash, 1 small yellow onion (chopped), 3 cups chicken broth, 3 tbsp. olive oil, 1/2 tsp. cumin powder, 2 carrots (chopped), 2 tsp. cinnamon powder, 1 and 1/2 tsp. Himalayan sea salt, 2 tbsp. ghee, and 1 tsp. chili powder.

Pre-heat the oven to about 400 degrees F. In a large bowl, combine the butternut squash, 1/2 tsp. salt, 1 tsp. cinnamon, olive oil, and 1/2 tsp. cumin. Coat the squash and mix together; spread mixture on a rimmed baking sheet. Toss the onion, apple slices and carrots to coat. Place on a rimmed baking sheet and roast 40 minutes, until soft. In a large pot, heat the ghee, add the roasted ingredients, chicken broth, and add 1 teaspoon each of chili powder, salt and cinnamon. Bring it to a boil, reduce the heat and simmer for 20 minutes. In a food processor, blend the ingredients until smooth; serve warm.

#287 White and Red Tomato-Onion Soup

4 large ripe tomatoes, 5 garlic cloves, 1/2 medium yellow onion, pepper (to taste), 1 tablespoon olive oil, 1 tablespoon chopped parsley, 1 1/2 cups almond milk, and 2 tablespoons tomato paste.

Directions: on a rimmed baking sheet, spread tomatoes and onions. Add pepper, olive oil, and chopped parsley; toss with your hands. Tuck the garlic cloves into the tomato to prevent from burning. Roast tomatoes for 40 minutes at 350 degrees F. In a large pot, add the almond milk and tomato paste. Add the ingredients into the pot and simmer for about 10 minutes. Add water if the creamy soup gets too thick; season with pepper to taste.

#288 Turkey, Black Bean and Kidney Chili Soup

1 can black beans, 2 cans of kidney beans, 2 1/2 tablespoons chili powder, 1/2 teaspoon crushed red pepper flakes, 1 can of tomato paste, 1 cup tomato juice, 1 small sweet onion, 1/2 teaspoon black pepper, 2 1/2 cups of water, 1 lb. lean ground turkey, and 1 diced tomatoes.

In a skillet, add onions and turkey; cook until meat is done. Transfer the cooked turkey, onions and the rest of the ingredients in a slow cooker. Cook on low heat for about 6 hours. Serve the soup in a bowl and garnish with diced onions parmesan cheese.

#289 Hot Black Beans and Kidney Chicken Soup

Variation #1; replace turkey with chicken.

#290 True Love's Beans

1 and 1/3 cups fried onions, 4 cups cooked cut green beans, 1/4 cup chopped red pepper, a dash of ground black pepper, 1/2 cup milk, and 1 can mushroom soup. Preheat your oven to 350 degrees F.

In a casserole, stir in the milk, black pepper, beans, 2/3 cups of onions and mushroom soup. Bake for 25 minutes and add the remaining onions; bake for 5 minutes more until the onions turn golden brown.

#291 Cucumber, Tomato, with Mango Cold Soup

4 tomatoes, 1/2 medium white onion, 1 clove garlic, lemon juice to taste, 1 cucumber, 1 tablespoon virgin olive oil, 1 red bell pepper, 1 scallion, 4 tablespoon freshly chopped cilantro, and 1/4 cup mango.

In a blender, add all the ingredients and puree; use a vegetable press to strain the cucumber pits and skin. Serve in a bowl and drizzle olive oil, sprinkle chopped scallions, mango and cilantro.

#292 Tomato Soup in Creamy Almond Milk

4 large ripe tomatoes, 5 garlic cloves, 1/2 medium yellow onion, 1 tablespoon olive oil, 1 tablespoon chopped parsley, 1 and 1/2 cups almond milk, 2 tablespoons tomato paste, and pepper to taste.

In a rimmed baking sheet, spread tomatoes and onions. Drizzle with the salt, pepper, olive oil, and chopped parsley. With your hands, toss the vegetables gently. Tuck garlic cloves into the tomato to prevent from burning. Roast in an oven for 40 minutes at 350 degrees F; remove and cool. In a large pot, add the almond milk and tomato paste. Add the ingredients into the pot and simmer for about 10 minutes.

#293 Bacon, Kale and Butternut Squash Soup

½ lb. bacon, 1/2 teaspoon paprika (smoked), 2 tablespoon bacon fat, 1 small cubed butternut squash, 1 1/2 tablespoon minced fresh sage, 16 oz. chopped frozen kale, and 4 cup water.

In a large Dutch oven, heat 1 tablespoon of bacon fat and cook stew bacon until it turns into golden brown. Add 1 tablespoon bacon of fat, smoked paprika, and sage; frequently stir the mixture to prevent it from burning. Add the kale, butternut squash and water to the pot. Bring to a boil and simmer for 1 hour before serving.

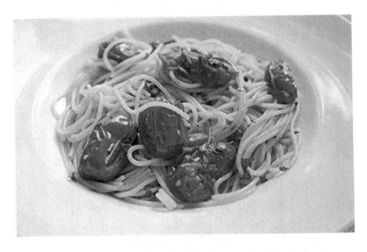

Category: Pasta; Recipes 294-325

Unless stated that it is to be baked, boil water in a pot; add pasta and cook al dente. In a slow-cooker, add all ingredients together. Cook for 4 hours on high heat. Toss with pasta and serve.

#294 Chicken Sausage with Spinach and Chili Flakes Pasta

2 cups spinach, 1/2 tsp. red chili flakes, 1/4 cup ricotta cheese, 1 lb. chicken sausage, 1/2 cup cooked whole-wheat spaghetti, and 1/3 cup tomato sauce.

#295 Mediterranean Pasta in Anchovies, Capers and Olives

To make this delicious recipe, you will need 1 lb. spaghetti pasta, ½ cup white wine, 1 can Italian tomatoes (crushed), ½ cup fresh basil (chopped), ½ tsp. red pepper flakes, 2 tbsp. capers, 3 tbsp.

olive oil, ½ tsp. black pepper, 1 small onion, 2 garlic cloves, 4 anchovy fillet, and ½ cup black olives.

#296 Pollo Arrabiata with Rigatoni Noodles

To prepare an intense Mediterranean meal, you need 1 and ½ lb. skinless chicken thighs, 1 jar Arrabiata pasta sauce, 1 lb. Rigatoni pasta, and grated parmesan cheese (topping).

#297 Shrimps and Tomatoes in Zucchini Noodles

You will need 6 medium plum tomatoes, 16 fresh asparagus, 1 tablespoon olive oil, 1/4 cup dry white wine, 4 cloves garlic, 1/4 cup fresh basil, 1/2 lb. shrimps, 1 tablespoon ghee, and 1 lb. zucchini noodles.

#298 Shrimp and Sausage Pasta with Mustard Dip

1 tablespoon and 1 teaspoon green onions, 2 tablespoons and 2 teaspoons fresh mushrooms, 1/4 pound medium shrimps, 1/4 teaspoon Worcestershire sauce, 2/3 cup heavy cream, 2 tablespoons and 2 teaspoons white wine, 1 and 1/2 teaspoons coarse grained mustard (store-bought), pepper to taste, 1 and 1/2 teaspoons garlic, 1 package angel hair pasta, and 4 links Andouille sausage.

#299 Baked Italian Sausage and Kale Lasagna

You need 3 bunches kale leaves, 1 lb. ziti pasta, 2 cups mozzarella cheese, red pepper flakes (to taste), 1 lb. ground spicy Italian sausage, 1 cup parmesan cheese, and 4 cloves garlic.

In a large pot, bring water to a rolling boil and add the ziti pasta. In a medium-sized pan, add olive oil and sauté the garlic and ground sausages until it turns brown. Once done, add in the kale leaves and cook until the leaves wilt. In a baking dish, add the ziti pasta and mix the sausage mixture.

Top the first layer with parmesan cheese. Seal top layer with mozzarella cheese and bake for 25 minutes at 375 degrees F.

#299 Tomatoes and Asparagus Linguini

This recipe will require you 6 medium plum tomatoes, 16 fresh asparagus, 1 tablespoon olive oil, 4 cloves garlic, 1/4 cup dry white wine, 1 tablespoon butter, 1 package linguini pasta, and 1/4 cup chopped basil leaves

#300 Shrimp and Kalamata Olives Pasta

4 cups whole grain angel hair pasta, 1/4 tsp. freshly ground black pepper, 1 lb. medium shrimp, 1/3 cup Kalamata olives, 1/4 cup fresh basil, 2 cups plum tomato, 2 tbsp. tablespoons capers, 2 garlic cloves, 1/4 cup crumbled feta cheese, 2 tsp. olive oil, and cooking spray.

#301 Beef Meatballs and Pasta

1 jar beef gravy, 1 container sour cream, and 1 bag beef meatballs

#302 Lamb Meatballs and Pasta

Variation #1; replace turkey with lamb.

#303 Chicken Meatballs and Pasta

Variation #2; replace turkey with chicken.

#304 Turkey Meatballs and Pasta

Variation #3; replace turkey with turkey.

#305 Pesto Tortellini with Broccoli

1 cup heavy cream, ¼ cup pesto (bottled), ¼ cup parmesan cheese, 12 ounces tortellini pasta, and 1 cups broccoli (steamed).

In a large pot, bring water to a boil then add the broccoli and tortellini pasta. Cook the vegetables for about 15 minutes until the broccoli is tender and pasta is al dente. In a saucepan, simmer the pesto sauce and a cup of heavy cream; stir until thickened. Remove from the heat and dust parmesan cheese on top before tossing with pasta and broccoli. Serve the pesto tortellini with garlic bread on the side and enjoy!

#306 Pesto Tortellini with Cauliflower

Variation #1; replace broccoli with 1 cup cauliflower.

#307 Garlic-Broccoli Rigatoni Pasta

1 cup broccoli florets, 2 tsp. garlic (minced), 2 tbsp. Parmesan cheese, 2 tsp. olive oil, 1/3 lb. rigatoni noodles, and black pepper (freshly ground).

#308 Garlic-Cauliflower Rigatoni Pasta

Variation #1; replace broccoli with 1 cup cauliflower.

#309 Garlic-Asparagus Rigatoni Pasta

Variation #1; replace broccoli with 1 asparagus bunch.

#310 Cheesy Asparagus and Tomato Primavera

1 bunch asparagus, 12 small cherry tomatoes, 3 carrots, 1 sweet red pepper, 1 sweet yellow pepper, 2 tablespoons olive oil, 2 tablespoons grated Parmesan, 3 cloves garlic, 1 lb. penne pasta, 1/4 teaspoon black pepper, and ½ cup yogurt.

#311 Cheesy Zucchini and Tomato Primavera

Variation #1; replace asparagus with 1 zucchini.

#312 Tomatoes and Basil Squash Pasta

First you need 3 pieces of large squash. For the tomato sauce, you will need 1/2 bunch fresh basil, 1/4 cup onion, 6 large tomatoes, 2 garlic cloves, 4 pieces of pitted dates, 1/2 cup cold-pressed olive oil, 5 sun-dried tomatoes, and 1/4 cup lemon juice.

For the squash "pasta" strands, use a potato peeler to peel the squash; create thin strands with a fork. In a bowl, add the squash strands and olive oil; set aside. For the sauce, put all the ingredients in a blender and puree until creamy. Place the squash strands on a plate and pour the creamy sauce on top. Garnish with tomatoes, olives and onions; serve and enjoy!

#313 Classic Aglio e Olio Spaghetti

6 garlic cloves, ½ cup Parmesan cheese (freshly grated), ½ cup extra-virgin olive oil, 1 lb. spaghetti, red pepper flakes to taste, and ground pepper to taste as well.

#314 All-Time Tomato, Olive and Caper Linguini

1 lb. linguine, 1 cup Italian parsley, 1 can of crushed tomatoes, ½ cup green olives, 2 cans anchovy fillets, 1 tsp. dried oregano, ½ tsp. hot pepper flakes, 2 tbsp. capers, ½ cup black olives, 2 tbsp. virgin olive oil, and 4 garlic cloves.

In a pot, boil salted water and add the pasta; cook for 15 minutes until al dente. In a food processor, pulse the tomatoes until crushed; set aside.

#315 Italian Sausages in Tomato-Basil over Squash Pasta

1 medium squash spaghetti, 1 lb. Italian sausage (crumbled), 1 can of tomato sauce, 2 tbsp. pepper relish (hot), 6 garlic cloves (whole), 2 tbsp. olive oil , 2 tsp. dried basil, and parsley for garnishing.

In a pot, bring salted water to a boil and add the squash spaghetti. In a colander, drain the liquid and set the pasta aside. In a large slow cooker, add and stir the olive oil, garlic, tomato sauce, seasoning and pepper relish. Cut the squash in halves, take out the seeds and place them face down in the cooker. Roll the ground sausage into small meatballs; add to the marinara sauce. In a slow cooker, cook the meatballs and sauce for five hours. Add meat and sauce over the spaghetti and garnish with parsley.

#316 Baked Cremini Mushrooms and Sausage-Crusted Mascarpone

1/2 pound sweet Italian sausage, 2 1/2 tbsp. Marsala wine, 16 Cremini mushrooms, 5 tbsp. olive oil, 1 cup breadcrumbs, 6 scallions, 5 ounces mascarpone cheese, 2 1/2 tbsp. parsley leaves, 2 garlic cloves, 1/2 cup Parmesan cheese, and Kosher salt to taste.

In a shallow bowl, add whole mushroom caps, Marsala wine and olive oil. Line the mushrooms in a greased baking dish and bake for 50 minutes at 325 degrees F. Once the stuffing turns golden brown, turn off heat; serve right away.

#317 Italian Spicy Sausage Pasta

1 lb. spicy Italian sausage, 1 package spaghetti, 1 can diced tomatoes, 1 onion, 1 tsp. dried basil, 1 package frozen spinach, 1 tbsp. olive oil, 4 cloves garlic, 1/2 cup Parmesan cheese, and 1 can chicken broth.

#318 Mediterranean Baked Beef Ravioli Lasagna

1 lb. ground beef, 1 jar spaghetti sauce, 1 package Ravioli, and 1 and 1/2 cups Mozzarella cheese. In a medium skillet, cook the ground beef over a medium to high heat. Grease a baking dish with olive oil and layer it with 1/2 ravioli, 1/3 pasta sauce, 1/2 cheese and 1/4 beef.

Repeat layering the skillet with the proportions and top the skillet with the remaining spaghetti sauce and the Mozzarella cheese. Cover the skillet and bake it in the oven for 45 minutes at 400 degrees F. As soon as the cheese melts, remove from the oven and serve.

#319 Baked 3 Cheese Ravioli Casserole

3 and 1/2 cups spaghetti sauce, 1/4 cup Parmesan cheese, 1 package cheese ravioli (24 pieces)., 4 cups Mozzarella cheese, and 2 cups Cottage cheese.

In a baking dish, lay 12 pieces of ravioli pasta on the base and pour 3 cups spaghetti sauce. Top with a cup of cottage cheese, and 2 cups of Mozzarella cheese. Add another layer of cheese ravioli on top and place baking dish in the oven. Bake for 40 minutes at 350 degrees F until the cheese melts; serve right away.

#320 Deep-Fried Breaded Ravioli

1 cup buttermilk, 1 jar marinara sauce (store bought), 2 cups bread crumbs (Panko), olive oil, 1/4 cup Parmesan cheese, and 1 box cheese ravioli (24 pieces).

Heat a frying pan to 325 degrees F and our olive oil with a depth of 2 inches. Prepare a small bowl to pour buttermilk and a plate to add the breadcrumbs. Dip the ravioli pasta in the buttermilk bowl then dredge on a plate of breadcrumbs. Fry the ravioli in a pan for three minutes; transfer to a plate lined with a paper towel. In a small bowl, add the warm marinara sauce for dipping. Garnish the ravioli with Parmesan cheese and dig in.

#321 Vegetarian Ravioli Alfredo with Mushrooms

4 cloves garlic, 2 tbsp. Parmesan cheese, 2 green onions, 3 tbsp. unsalted butter, 1 package frozen cheese ravioli, 1 package

mushrooms, 1/4 tsp. red pepper flakes, 1 container Alfredo sauce, and 5 cups water

#322 Fried Cracker Crumbs Ravioli with Marinara Dip

1 tsp. Italian seasoning, 1 1/2 cups marinara sauce (for dipping), 2 tbsp. almond milk, 1/2 tsp. garlic powder, 20 unsalted cheese crackers, 3 tbsp. Parmesan cheese, 1 package frozen cheese ravioli, 3 cups vegetable oil , 1/4 tsp. black pepper, parsley for garnishing, and 1 egg.

Preheat your oven to 325 degrees F. In a medium frying pan, pour vegetable oil at around 2 inches deep. Pulse the cheese crackers in a food processor until they turn into cracker crumbs. Prepare the pasta by filling a shallow-bottomed dish with pepper, garlic powder, parmesan cheese and Italian seasoning. In a small bowl, beat one egg and our 2 tablespoons of milk. Dip each of the 24 pieces of Ravioli into egg wash then dredge on the plate of cracker crumbs. Drop the ravioli pasta in the frying pan and deep-fry for a minute; reversing from side to side for an even fry. Transfer cooked ravioli on a paper towel to absorb excess oil. Once all the ravioli pasta is cooked, top it with Parmesan Cheese. Serve the Marinara Dip and enjoy.

#323 Cheesy Half Hour Baked Ravioli

1/2 cup Parmesan cheese, 1 jar spaghetti sauce, 1 package frozen cheese ravioli, 3 ounces sliced pepperoni, 1/2 cup Mozzarella cheese, and water.

In a large pot, add the frozen ravioli pasta and fill it with water. Boil the pasta for 15 minutes, drain the water and set aside. In a glass dish, pour half of the jar of spaghetti sauce, top with pepperoni slices and parmesan cheese. Layer in the cooked cheese ravioli and pour the remaining spaghetti sauce and add ½ cup of

Mozzarella cheese on top. Bake in the oven for 30 minutes at 350 degrees F; serve with extra slices of pepperoni.

#324 Breaded Italian Meat Ravioli

You will need 1 package frozen cheese ravioli, 1/4 cup water, 2 eggs, 1 cup flour, ½ cup marinara sauce, 1 cup breadcrumbs, and 1 tsp. Italian seasoning.

Thaw the cheese ravioli at room temperature and set aside. In a small bowl, whisk two eggs for the Ravioli wash. Use a shallow dish to combine Italian seasoning, garlic salt, flour and plain breadcrumbs. Dip the cheese ravioli in the egg wash, dredge in the breadcrumb mixture and deep fry. In a small sauce dish, pour a half cup of warm marinara sauce to dip the breaded pasta bite.

#325 Herbed Beef Ravioli in Mozzarella

To prepare this recipe, you will need 1 tbsp. dried basil, 1 cup mozzarella cheese, 1 bag beef ravioli, 1 jar pasta sauce, 1 cup water, 1 tsp. dried thyme, 1 can tomato sauce, 1 tsp. dried oregano, ½ tsp. red chili peppers, and 1 tsp. dried rosemary.

In a slow-cooker, add beef ravioli, rosemary, basil, thyme, oregano, ½ pasta sauce, red pepper and tomato sauce. Cook the ravioli for 4 hours until it absorbed all the flavors of the sauce. Serve on a plate and top with Parmesan cheese.

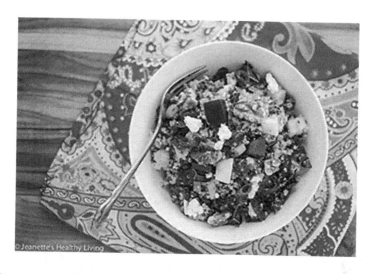

Category: Quinoa Soups and salad, Recipes #326-330

#326 Mediterranean Quinoa Soup in Zucchini and Tomatoes

1 tbsp. lemon juice (freshly squeezed), 2 tbsp. olive oil, 1 cup zucchini, 3 cups water, 1 tsp. ground coriander, 1 tsp. dried oregano, 1 cup diced potatoes, ½ tsp. ground pepper, 1 ½ cup fresh tomatoes, 2 cups onions, ½ cup raw quinoa, 1 tsp. Himalayan sea salt, 1 cup red bell peppers (chopped), and 1 tsp. ground cumin.

In a pot, heat olive oil and add salt and onions over medium heat. In a small bowl, rinse the quinoa rice; place a mesh strainer on top to drain the quinoa. Once drained, transfer quinoa to the pot and combine with oregano, bell pepper, potatoes, cumin, water, coriander and tomatoes. Bring to a boil for around 10 minutes. Add lemon juice and zucchini in the pot and simmer for 20 minutes until all the vegetables become tender.

#327 Quinoa and Walnut-Pea Soup

To make a feel good low carb Mediterranean soup, you need 1 1/2 cups frozen peas, 2 cups water, 1 small onion, 1 cup quinoa, 1/2 tsp. Himalayan sea salt, 1 tbsp. olive oil, 2 tbsp. walnuts (chopped), and 1/4 tsp. pepper.

In a saucepan, cook the quinoa with water and simmer it for 15 minutes until fluffy. In a small skillet, sauté onions and add the peas; season with Himalayan sea salt, and pepper. Add the pea mixture with the cooked quinoa. Serve this dish with the remaining chopped walnuts and enjoy hot.

#328 Quinoa Greek Salad in Cucumber and Olives

2 cups chicken stock, 1 cup quinoa, 1/2 cup red pepper, 1/2 cup green pepper, 1/2 cup cucumber, 1/4 cup green onion, 1/4 cup black olives, and 3 ounces feta cheese. For the salad dressing, you need 1/4 cup lemon juice, 2 tbsp. olive oil, 1 tsp. minced garlic, 1/2 tsp. basil, 1/2 tsp. dried oregano, and pepper to taste.

In a saucepan, add chicken stock and bring to a boil. Add in the quinoa, cook for 15 minutes; add feta cheese and vegetables. To prepare the dressing, whisk the olive oil, pepper, basil, lemon juice, garlic, oregano and Himalayan salt in a bowl. Serve the salad right away and enjoy!

#329 Spicy Black Bean- Quinoa Salad with Steamed Broccoli

For this Mediterranean quinoa salad, you need 4 tsp. fresh lime juice, 1/4 tsp. ground cumin, 1 tsp. olive oil, 1 tbsp. chopped cilantro, pepper and Himalayan sea salt to taste, 2 tsp. jalapeno chili, 1 can black beans, 1 cup quinoa, 1 cup bell pepper, 1 cup water, 1/4 tsp. ground coriander, 2 tbsp. minced scallions, and 2 cups chopped tomatoes.

In a small pot, bring water to a rolling boil and the quinoa. In a medium-sized bowl, combine the cumin, oil, cilantro, lime juice, and scallions. Once the quinoa is cooked, serve on a plate and add steamed broccoli florets on top.

#330 Baked Egg Basket over Green Bells and Quinoa

1 can of tomatoes, 1/8 teaspoon paprika, 1/8 teaspoon rosemary, 1 garlic clove, minced, olive oil (for frying), 8 egg yolks, 1 soft boiled egg, 1 medium green pepper, 1/4 cup butter, ground black pepper (to taste), 1 large onion, 2 cups quinoa.

In a medium-sized pan, place a small glass bowl with 8 beaten egg yolks and 1 egg; bake in the oven for 25 minutes at low heat, slice in squares. In a skillet, sauté the pepper, garlic, rosemary, onion and paprika with butter. Add the sliced eggs and tomatoes together with its liquid; cook for 10 minutes. To serve, spoon the eggs over brown rice and sprinkle pepper to taste.

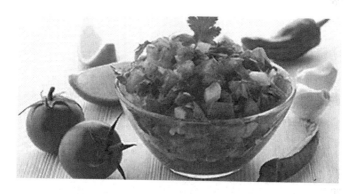

Category: Salsa; Recipes #331-338

Note: Dinner will not be complete without a simple but delicious dip called the salsa. It brings an extra oomph to grilled fish, meat and turkey. Salads can conclude a meal but if you bring out the pitas or unsalted cracker, the salsa will definitely lighten up the meal.

#331 Cider Vinegar Dressing in Thyme and Cayenne

½ cup salad oil, 1 tbsp. cider vinegar, 1 tbsp. Dijon mustard, 1 tbsp. water, 1 tsp. thyme, 1 tsp. onion powder, 1 tsp. garlic powder , and 1 tsp. cayenne pepper.

In a glass jar, combine the salad oil, cider vinegar, mustard, sugar, water, thyme, onion powder, garlic powder and cayenne pepper. Shake the ingredients for the dressing and drizzle on the chicken with mix greens.

#332 Fresh Salsa Dip in Cilantro and Tomatoes

1/4 cup green sweet pepper, 1/4 cup red onion, 2 tomatoes, 1/2 teaspoon minced garlic, 3 teaspoons cilantro, black pepper, and hot pepper sauce (for added flavor).

In a medium bowl, add the minced red onions, tomatoes, garlic, cilantro and drop of hot sauce. Combine the ingredients together to make a salsa and chill for 30 minutes before serving.

#333 Tomatillo and Cumin Salsa

2 tsp. cumin seeds, 1 jalapeño (chopped), 1 small onion, 3 cloves garlic, 1/2 cup cilantro (chopped) 1 1/2 tsp. cane sugar, and 1 pound tomatillos.

In a medium-sized saucepan, boil the onions, jalapeño, tomatillos and water then bring to a simmer for about 8 minutes. Transfer the cooked vegetables to a processor and blend. In a small skillet, add the cumin seeds and toast for 2 minutes. Add the powdered cumin seeds, cane sugar and cilantro in a blender and puree until smooth.

#334 Jalapeño-Tomato Salsa with Cucumber

To make this mouthwatering salsa, you will need 1 lb. tomatoes, 1/2 cup sweet onion, 1/2 cup cilantro, 1 small jalapeño, 2 tbsp.

fresh lime juice, ground pepper to taste, and 1 large cucumber (seedless).

In a bowl, toss the chopped tomatoes, cilantro, jalapeños, lime juice and season with pepper. Serve the salsa with tortilla chips and enjoy!

#335 Fresh Tomato, Garlic, Chili and Cilantro Salsa

3 large tomatoes, 1 clove garlic, 4 green onions, 2 tbsp. purple onions, 3 jalapeños, 2 tbsp. chopped cilantro, and 2 tbsp. lime juice.

On a chopping board, chop 3 large tomatoes, green onions, purple onions, jalapeños then mince garlic and cilantro leaves. In a blender, combine all the ingredients, pulse for 10 seconds.

#336 Chili Bell Peppers and Arugula Salsa

3 garlic cloves, ground black pepper to taste, 2 tbsp. chopped arugula leaves, 1 large bell pepper, 1/4 tsp. red chili flakes, 2 tbsp. apple cider vinegar, 6 chopped green onions, and 2 tbsp. olive oil.

In a small bowl, add garlic cloves, bell pepper, green onions, arugula, chili flakes, vinegar, pepper, and olive oil. Mix all the ingredients together and toss to blend well with the spices.

#337 Cranberry and Jalapeño Salsa

2 green onions (chopped), 1/2 apple (chopped), 1 1/2 cups frozen cranberries, 1/2 jalapeño, 2 tbsp. chopped cilantro, 4 tbsp. cane sugar, 1 tbsp. lemon juice, and 1 tbsp. minced ginger.

In a blender, add the apple, cranberries, green onions, chili, sugar, ginger, cilantro, and lime juice in a food processor, set to pulse for 30 seconds.

#338 Spicy Cilantro Salsa with Kumquats and Onions

1/4 tsp. red pepper flakes, 1/2 cup red onion (chopped), 1/4 cup fresh cilantro (chopped)

2 cups kumquats, kosher salt, 3 tbsp. olive oil, and cayenne pepper to taste.

On a chopping board, chop the kumquats, red onion and cilantro leaves. In a large bowl, mix the chopped vegetables; add red pepper flakes, olive oil, cayenne pepper and kosher salt.

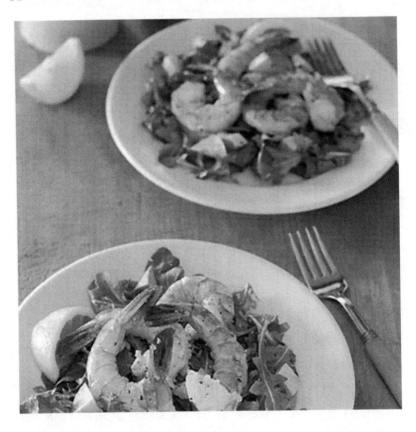

Category: Seafood; Recipes #339-353

#340 Peppered Shrimp, Cilantro and Tomato

You will need 1 teaspoon chopped garlic, 1 pound medium shrimp, 2 tablespoons olive oil, 1/2 teaspoon ground cumin, 1/8 teaspoon crushed red pepper, 1/8 teaspoon black pepper, juice of 1 lime, 1 chopped tomato, and 1/2 cup chopped cilantro.

To prepare the recipe cook the deveined, peeled shrimps, garlic, and olive oil in a pan. Add ground cumin, red pepper and black pepper; gently mix. Drizzle freshly squeezed lime juice; add tomatoes and cilantro.

#341 Tuna Pita Pockets with Romaine Lettuce

For this recipe, you will need 1/2 cup green bell peppers (finely chopped), 3/4 cup diced tomatoes, 1 1/2 cups romaine lettuce, 1/2 cup broccoli (finely chopped), 1/2 cup shredded carrots, 2 cans white tuna in water (low-salt), 1/4 cup onion (finely chopped), 3 pita pockets (whole-wheat) and 1/2 cup ranch dressing (low-fat).

To make it, add the tomatoes, carrots, lettuce, broccoli, peppers, and onions; toss everything in a large bowl. In a small bowl, combine the ranch dressing, tuna mixture and lettuce. Scoop the tuna salad and fill each pita pocket; serve immediately.

#342 Moroccan Shrimp with Arugula and Coriander

This yummy dish yields 1/4 cup fresh lemon juice, 4 cups baby arugula, 1/2 cup cane sugar, 3/4 tsp. ground cumin, 1/4 tsp. ground cinnamon, cayenne powder (to taste), 3/4 tsp. ground coriander, 1 lb. large shrimp, and 1 1/2 tbsp. olive oil.

Directions are as follows. In a shallow pot, boil the lemon juice, cane sugar for 45 minutes. Heat a grill pan and shrimp and cook 2 then top it with arugula; remove and transfer to a medium-bowl.

Now toss the cooked shrimp with coriander, cinnamon, cumin and olive oil. Once the shrimp mixture is fully coated, toss the arugula, olive oil and lemon juice. Transfer the shrimps on a plate and serve.

#343 Moroccan Shrimp with Romaine Lettuce and Coriander

Variation #1; replace arugula with 1 head of lettuce.

#344 Moroccan Shrimp with Cabbage and Coriander

Variation #2; replace arugula with 1 head of cabbage.

#345 Hot Grits with Cajun-Style Shrimps

1/2 cup green onions (sliced), 1 cup onion (chopped), 1 cup milk (fat-free), 1 teaspoon Cajun seasoning, and 36 pieces medium shrimps, 1 minced garlic clove. 1 tablespoon olive oil, ½ cup ounces minced Tasso ham, 1 cup quick-cooking grits (uncooked), 2 1/4 cups water, 1 tablespoon butter (unsalted), and 1 cup shredded sharp cheddar cheese.

In a large skillet, heat olive oil and sauté the minced Tasso ham, garlic and onions. Add the shrimps and Cajun seasoning and cook for 2 minutes. Add ¼ cup of water and stir in the butter. Remove the shrimps and ham mixture from the skillet and transfer to a plate. In the same skillet, boil the milk, and 2 cups of water; reduce heat before adding the grits. Cook the grits for 5 minutes; remove pan from heat and add the cheese. Serve the hot grits on a plate and top with the ham mixture, green onions and shrimps.

#346 Pan-Fried Scallops with Roasted Squash and Kale

2 tsp. lemon juice, 2 cups kale, 3 ounces of scallops, 2 tsp. canola oil, 1 1/2 cups squash (roasted), and 1/2 teaspoon ground sage.

In a large skillet, cook the scallops in canola oil for about 2 minutes. Flip the scallops to the other side and cook for another minute; remove from the skillet and set aside. In the same skillet, sauté the kale leaves and squash. Drizzle lemon juice and season with ground sage. Add a dash of pepper to taste.

#347 Pan-Fried Scallops with Roasted Squash and Arugula

Variation #1; replace kale with 2 cups arugula leaves.

#348 Shrimp Rolls in Brown Rice

You will need 1 cup palm oil, 2 small peppers, 3 cups rice flour, 1 large onion, and 1 cup shrimps.

In a bowl, mix the rice flour and water to form a thick paste; set aside. Chop the onions and add the pepper; grind together. Combine the onion mixture with the rice mixture and add the shrimps. Cut the fire-heated banana leaves into small squares to wrap the rice and shrimp mixture. Place the banana leaves on a baking tray and place it in steamer for about an hour. Serve and consume right away.

#349 Black-eyed Beans with Fried Plantains and Shrimp

You will need 1 pint of vegetable cooking oil, 1 cup shrimps 1 egg, 2 cups black-eyed beans, 1 large pepper, and 1 small onion.

In a small bowl, soak the pre-washed black-eyed beans for about 2 hours. Transfer the beans into a mortar and grind to a paste. Remove the bean paste and place into a medium-sized bowl. Add chopped pepper and onions into the beans mixture and use a hand-held mixer; add in the egg. In a pan, pour the oil and deep-fry the bean mixture and shrimps until it turns golden brown.

#350 Lentils with Fried Plantains and Shrimp

Variation #1; replace Black-eyed beans with 2 cups lentils.

#351 Pinto Beans with Fried Plantains and Shrimp

Variation #2; replace Black-eyed beans with 2 cups pinto beans.

#352 Brazilian Stew in Spicy Shrimp

¼ cup red pepper (roasted), ¼ cup fresh cilantro, 1 clove garlic, 1½ lbs. shrimp, 2 tbsp. lime juice (freshly squeezed), ¼ cup olive oil, 1 can diced tomato, 2 tbsp. hot sauce, 1 cup coconut milk, ¼ cup onion, pepper (to taste), and 6 bowls of risotto.

In a pan, add olive oil and sauté the chopped onions, red peppers and garlic. Add in the cilantro, shrimp, tomatoes, hot sauce and coconut milk. Heat to a rolling boil and add pepper and lime juice to taste. Add a bowl of risotto and serve stew in ceramic bowls; garnish with extra cilantro.

#353 Mediterranean Spicy Curry Quinoa with Garbanzo and Pine Nuts

You will need 1 cup quinoa, 1/2 cup toasted pine nuts, 1 small onion, 1/2 cup raisins, 1/2 tsp. black pepper, 1 tbsp. olive oil, 1 can of garbanzo beans, 1/2 tsp. ground cumin, 1/2 tsp. Himalayan sea salt, 1 1/2 cups chicken stock, 1 1/2 tsp. curry powder, 1/4 tsp. cinnamon, and 1 clove garlic.

In a saucepan, cook the garlic and onions in olive oil then stir in the salt, cumin, cinnamon, chicken stock, curry powder and pepper. Add the quinoa to the mixture and boil for 20 minutes; check if the quinoa has absorbed the liquid. Add the garbanzo beans, raisins and pine nuts on top. Serve right away to enjoy.

Remove from the oven and sprinkle cheddar cheese on top. Pop it back in the oven and bake for 40 minutes to melt the cheese and wilt the spinach leaves.

Chapter 4

Mediterranean Low-Carb Snack Recipes

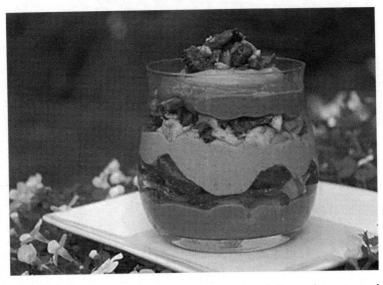

Here are after meal recipes that taste as good as the most sinful desserts you can ever imagine. What is the secret behind these explosive flavors? Well, it's for you to find out!

Category: Low-Carb Snacks on the Go; Recipes #354

#354 Zucchini Fritters with Feta in Yogurt Dip

Veggies and feta cheese in one recipe? Make your Mediterranean feast by using 2 and 1/2 lb. zucchini, 2 oz. feta cheese, 2 eggs; 3

tbsp. fresh mint, 1/4 cup yogurt (for dipping), 1/2 cup frying oil, 3 garlic cloves, 2 tbsp. flour and pepper (to taste).

Make the fritters by dry the zucchini and shred them. In a bowl, mix flour, garlic, pepper, and eggs. Add mint, feta cheese and zucchini. In a pan, heat oil to fry zucchini batter; blot excess oil. Serve zucchini fritters on a plate with plain yogurt as dip.

#355 Cucumber Fritters with Feta in Yogurt Dip

Variation #1; replace zucchini with 1/2 lb. cucumbers.

#356 Cornmeal Crisps

Prepare 3/4 cup fat-free milk, 3/4 cup water, 1/4 cup oil, 1 teaspoon baking powder, 2 cups yellow cornmeal and confectioner's sugar (for dusting).

All you have to do is mix ¼ cup of oil and add the milk, water, baking powder and cornmeal in a bowl. Pour the batter in a hot iron skillet and cook on low heat for 15 minutes. Once the cornmeal crisps are done, dust confectioner's sugar on top and serve on a plate.

#357 Crusted Cornmeal Couches

You need 2 eggs, 4 cups corn meal, 2 teaspoons baking powder, 1/2 cup vegetable oil, and 1 tablespoon unsalted butter.

Begin by heating the oil in a pan. In a small bowl, moisten the cornmeal with warm water then add eggs and baking powder. Pour the cornmeal mixture into the hot lard. This mixture will enable you to form a crust. Cover the pan and wait until the crust is set. Remove from the pan and serve with a glass of milk on the side.

#358 Mediterranean Brown Rice Fritters

2 cups cooked brown rice, 2 eggs, 2 teaspoons baking powder, 3 tablespoons cane sugar, 1/4 teaspoon vanilla, 6 tablespoons almond flour, 4 cups cooking oil (for deep frying), and confectioner's sugar (for dusting).

Mix baking powder, eggs, brown rice, cane sugar, seasonings and almond flour in a bowl. Add oil in a deep-bottomed frying pan and drop several spoonful of the rice mixture; fry until golden brown. Drain the cooked fritters on paper towels and serve on a plate. Sprinkle with confectioner's sugar and eat right away.

#359 Fruit Cocktail Cake with Butter Icing

5 cups fruit cocktail juice, 2 eggs, 2 teaspoons baking soda, 2 cups flour, and 1 1/2 cups granulated sugar. You also need these ingredients to make the butter icing: 1 teaspoon vanilla, 1/2 cup milk, 3/4 cup sugar cane, and 1/2 cup butter.

Line a medium-sized baking pan with parchment paper. In a mixing bowl, mix the sugar cane, flour, fruit cocktail, cocktail juice, and baking soda. Mix all the ingredients until a batter is formed, pour into the greased pans. Bake the pans in the oven for about 35 minutes at 350 degrees F. Meanwhile, prepare the cake icing by combine vanilla, butter and milk in a saucepan. Bring the 4 ingredients to a gentle boil then once it is done, pour over the cake.

#360 Mandarin Oranges and Pineapple Cake

1 package instant vanilla pudding mix, 1 package frozen whipped topping, 1 can of mandarin oranges, 1 package yellow cake mix, and 1 can crushed pineapple (unsweetened).

Directions: preheat your oven to 350 degrees F. In two round pans, line them with parchment paper and set aside. In a medium-sized bowl, add one package instant vanilla pudding mix with pineapples, eggs and water; mix until smooth. Add all the oranges from the can; fold in the pudding mix batter. Divide the batter and pour into the lined round pans; bake in the oven for 30 minutes. Once the cakes are done, remove them from the pans and transfer to wire racks to cool down. Spread the whipped toppings on over the cakes and refrigerate for 30 minutes.

#361 Strawberry Carob with Almond-Vanilla Cream

For this recipe, you will need 1 cup almond milk, 3 large eggs, 1/2 teaspoon vanilla extract, and 1 cup strawberries.

To make the dish, get a pot, place the almond milk and gently simmer. In separate bowls, add egg yolks and egg white; beat separately until frothy. Add hot almond milk and vanilla extract to the tempered eggs; freeze for 2 hours. In a food processor, puree the sliced strawberries; add mixture with the chilled cream mixture, serve in a tall glass to enjoy.

#362 Almond and Vanilla Cream Blueberry Carob

Variation #1: replace strawberry with 1 cup of blueberries.

#363 Almond and Vanilla Cream Blackberry Carob

Variation #2: replace strawberry with 1 cup of blackberries.

#364 Almond and Vanilla Cream Cherry Carob

Variation #3: replace strawberry with 1 cup of cherries.

#365 Almond and Vanilla Cream Raspberry Carob

Variation #4: replace strawberry with 1 cup of raspberries.

Conclusion

I hope this book was able to help you sustain a low carb diet. Consider this diet as a long-term choice in order to keep your weight in check while eating the food you love.

365 different low carbohydrate recipes were given to you to have flavor variations. 90% of the time, dieters find it boring to keep on eating the same food. This is your chance to whip up mouthwatering meals that still have the same low-carb content you need.

Start preparing meals that will benefit you and your family's health. Isn't it amazing to be given a chance to plot different meals you can mix and match at any given day? If you enjoyed this book, then would you be kind enough to leave a review for this book on Amazon? It'd be greatly appreciated!

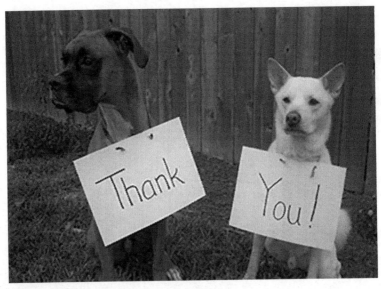

Thank you and good luck!

Made in the USA
Lexington, KY
26 December 2017